OAPL
OXFORD AMERICAN PAIN LIBRARY

Adjuvant Analgesics

This material is not intended to be, and should not be considered, a substitute for medical or other professional advice. Treatment for the conditions described in this material is highly dependent on the individual circumstances. While this material is designed to offer accurate information with respect to the subject matter covered and to be current as of the time it was written, research and knowledge about medical and health issues are constantly evolving, and dose schedules for medications are being revised continually, with new side effects recognized and accounted for regularly. Readers must therefore always check the product information and clinical procedures with the most up-to-date published product information and data sheets provided by the manufacturers and the most recent codes of conduct and safety regulation. Oxford University Press and the authors make no representations or warranties to readers, express or implied, as to the accuracy or completeness of this material, including without limitation that they make no representations or warranties as to the accuracy or efficacy of the drug dosages mentioned in the material. The authors and the publishers do not accept, and expressly disclaim, any responsibility for any liability, loss, or risk that may be claimed or incurred as a consequence of the use and/or application of any of the contents of this material.

The Publisher is responsible for author selection and the Publisher and the Author(s) make all editorial decisions, including decisions regarding content. The Publisher and the Author(s) are not responsible for any product information added to this publication by companies purchasing copies of it for distribution to clinicians.

OAPL
OXFORD AMERICAN PAIN LIBRARY

Adjuvant Analgesics

Edited by

David Lussier, MD

Assistant Professor of Medicine
Institut universitaire de gériatrie de Montréal
 University of Montréal
Division of Geriatric Medicine and Alan-Edwards
 Centre for Research in Pain
 McGill University
Montréal, Quebec, Canada

Pierre Beaulieu, MD, PhD

Associate Professor of Anesthesiology and Pharmacology
Faculty of Medicine
 University of Montréal
Centre hospitalier de l'Université de Montréal
 Montréal, Quebec, Canada

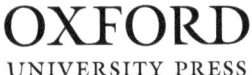

OXFORD
UNIVERSITY PRESS

Oxford University Press is a department of the University of
Oxford. It furthers the University's objective of excellence in research,
scholarship, and education by publishing worldwide.

Oxford   New York
Auckland   Cape Town   Dar es Salaam   Hong Kong   Karachi
Kuala Lumpur   Madrid   Melbourne   Mexico City   Nairobi
New Delhi   Shanghai   Taipei   Toronto

With offices in
Argentina   Austria   Brazil   Chile   Czech Republic   France   Greece
Guatemala   Hungary   Italy   Japan   Poland   Portugal   Singapore
South Korea   Switzerland   Thailand   Turkey   Ukraine   Vietnam

Oxford is a registered trademark of Oxford University Press
in the UK and certain other countries.

Published in the United States of America by
Oxford University Press
198 Madison Avenue, New York, NY 10016

© Oxford University Press 2015

All rights reserved. No part of this publication may be reproduced, stored in
a retrieval system, or transmitted, in any form or by any means, without the prior
permission in writing of Oxford University Press, or as expressly permitted by law,
by license, or under terms agreed with the appropriate reproduction rights organization.
Inquiries concerning reproduction outside the scope of the above should be sent to the
Rights Department, Oxford University Press, at the address above.

You must not circulate this work in any other form
and you must impose this same condition on any acquirer.

Library of Congress Cataloging-in-Publication Data
Adjuvant analgesics / volume editors, David Lussier and Pierre Beaulieu.
  p. ; cm. —(Oxford American Pain Library)
Includes bibliographical references.
ISBN 978–0–19–989181–8
I. Lussier, David, editor.   II. Beaulieu, Pierre, 1958– , editor.
III. Series: Oxford American Pain Library.
[DNLM: 1. Analgesics.   2. Chronic Pain—drug therapy. QV 95]
RM319
615.7′83—dc23
2014036646

Preface

From the use of opium poppy extracts and cannabis sativa millennia ago to the development of novel analgesics, our knowledge of the pharmacology of pain has evolved considerably. Most of this improved knowledge has occurred in the past few years. Indeed, improved understanding of the mechanisms of pain at cellular, molecular, and synaptic levels has allowed the development of analgesics acting on new targets, providing new hope for better pain management and improved quality of life in millions of patients worldwide.

There are many chapters and textbooks devoted to opioids but few on other analgesics, the so-called "adjuvant analgesics." These drugs include analgesic antidepressants and anticonvulsants that are recommended as first-line therapy for neuropathic pain (gabapentinoids, tricyclic antidepressants, duloxetine), cannabinoids, topical analgesics, local anesthetics, antihyperalgesics. We therefore felt that a new book was needed to fill a gap in the literature—a book that would offer a comprehensive review of the pharmacology of adjuvant analgesics that would be useful for clinicians and clinical researchers, either physicians or other health professionals. To facilitate use for clinical purposes, we also included chapters on clinical entities such as neuropathic pain, cancer pain, postoperative pain, and fibromyalgia.

Each chapter provides a detailed review of the current state of knowledge on a specific topic and offers a framework for considering future developments on that topic.

In preparing this book, we faced two main challenges. The first was to cover a very broad area but still provide detailed information on each topic for the practicing physician without exceeding a reasonable number of pages. The second challenge we encountered was to provide reviews that would still be timely after the book was published, given the rapid evolution of knowledge in this field. We are confident that we have succeeded in meeting both challenges, mainly because all chapters were authored by leading experts on the topic covered. We are very fortunate that we were able to include so many world-renowned experts on the pharmacology of pain in this book. We therefore extend our gratitude to all those who agreed to take up the challenge of providing this state-of-the-art review of such rapidly evolving fields. Our gratitude also goes to Andrea Knobloch and all the Oxford University Press staff, for their patience and help during the publication process. Finally, we thank Dr. Russell K. Portenoy, Editor of this Oxford Pain series, for his guidance throughout the process.

Contents

Contributors *ix*

1	**Overview of Pain Management** *David Lussier and Pierre Beaulieu*	**1**
2	**Classification of Analgesics** *David Lussier and Pierre Beaulieu*	**5**
3	**Antidepressants** *C. Peter N. Watson*	**11**
4	**Anticonvulsants** *David Lussier*	**21**
5	**Cannabinoids** *Julie Desroches and Pierre Beaulieu*	**33**
6	**Local Anesthetics** *Patrick Friederich*	**47**
7	**N-Methyl-D-aspartate Antagonists** *Philippe Richebé, Laurent Bollag, and Cyril Rivat*	**59**
8	**Topical Adjuvant Analgesics** *Jana Sawynok*	**71**
9.1	**Neuropathic Pain** *Nadine Attal*	**79**
9.2	**Cancer-related Pain** *Paul N. Luong and Russell K. Portenoy*	**95**
9.3	**Rheumatic Pain and Fibromyalgia** *Mary-Ann Fitzcharles*	**107**
9.4	**Acute Postoperative Pain** *Pierre Beaulieu*	**119**
10	**Drug-Drug Interactions of Adjuvant Analgesics** *David R. P. Guay*	**131**

Index *147*

Contributors

Nadine Attal, MD, PhD
INSERM U 987
Center for Evaluation and
Treatment of Pain
Hôpital Ambroise Paré, APH
Boulogne-Billancourt, France
University of Versailles
Saint-Quentin-en-Yvelines
Versailles, France

Laurent Bollag, MD
Associate Professor of
Anesthesiology and Pain Medicine
University of Washington
Seattle, Washington

Julie Desroches, PhD
Department of Pharmacology
Faculty of Medicine
University of Montreal
Montréal, Canada

Mary-Ann Fitzcharles, MB, ChB, FRCPC
Associate Professor of Medicine
Division of Rheumatology
McGill University; Alan Edwards
Pain Management Unit
McGill University Health Center
Montréal, Quebec, Canada

Patrick Friederich, MD
Professor and Chairman of
Anesthesiology
Department of Anaesthesiology,
Critical Care Medicine, Pain Therapy
Bogenhausen Hospital
Academic Hospital of Technische
Universität München
Munich, Germany

David R. P. Guay, PharmD, FCP, FCCP, FASCP
Professor Emeritus of Experimental
and Clinical Pharmacology
College of Pharmacy
University of Minnesota
Consultant Staff
HealthPartners Geriatrics
HealthPartners Inc.
Minneapolis, Minnesota

Paul N. Luong, MD
Lead Palliative Medicine Physician
Kaiser Permanente Central
Valley Area
Modesto, California

Russell K. Portenoy, MD
Executive Director
MJHS Institute for Innovation in
Palliative Care
Chief Medical Officer
MJHS Hospice and Palliative Care
New York, New York
Professor of Neurology
Albert Einstein College of Medicine
Bronx, New York

Philippe Richebé, MD, PhD
Professor of Anesthesiology
Department of Anesthesiology
University of Montreal
Maisonneuve-Rosemont Hospital
Montréal, Quebec, Canada

Cyril Rivat, PhD
Associate Professor
University of Montpellier
Institute of Neurosciences of
Montpellier (INM)-INSERM U1051
Saint Eloi Hospital
Montpellier, France

Jana Sawynok, PhD
Department of Pharmacology
Dalhousie University
Halifax, Nova Scotia, Canada

C. Peter N. Watson, MD, FRCPC
Assistant Professor of Medicine
University of Toronto
Toronto, Ontario, Canada

Chapter 1

Overview of Pain Management

David Lussier and Pierre Beaulieu

Pain, especially chronic persistent pain, is a multidimensional experience defined as "An unpleasant sensory and emotional experience associated with actual or potential tissue damage, or described in terms of such damage" [1]. As such, it responds better to a multimodal, multidimensional, interdisciplinary approach. Pain management should not only focus on decreasing the noxious stimuli but also address the multiple dimensions and aim to minimize impact on mood, function, and quality of life. To achieve these goals, treatment should combine nonpharmacological (physical, psychological), pharmacological, interventional, and specific approaches to pain management [2].

Nonpharmacological approaches to pain management

Nonpharmacological approaches are traditionally categorized as physical and psychological approaches.

Physical approaches include passive therapies such as transcutaneous electrical nerve stimulation, ultrasounds, massage, and shock-wave therapies. Although these therapies can usually provide some short-term relief, response is usually better and more sustained when active therapies are used, such as exercises (aimed at increasing strength, tone, or flexibility) and rehabilitation practices. When managing pain, the goal should always be to ensure that the patient has an active role and is fully involved in the therapeutic plan.

To achieve this goal, psychological approaches are used as an essential component of the pain-management strategy. Psychological approaches include cognitive-behavioral therapy, strategies based on emotional disclosure, and mind-body interventions (eg, yoga, mindfulness) [3]. The most appropriate strategy for a given patient can be determined based on the nature and characteristics of the patient's pain, comorbidities, personality traits, and previous response to other treatments.

Interventional approaches

Interventional approaches to pain management include various techniques aimed at reducing pain depending on the location and type of pain such as spinal blocks (epidural or facet), intra-articular blocks, peripheral nerve blocks, coeliac block, or sympathetic block. Invasive routes of delivery of analgesics, such as intrathecal, can also be used in patients who do not respond to conventional oral or transdermal routes.

Specific approaches

Rather than treating pain, it is preferable to treat the cause of the pain, whenever possible. For example, the following surgeries may be performed to treat pain: joint replacement in a patient with osteoarthritis, laminectomy and fusion for a patient with spinal stenosis, and gamma knife ablation for patients with trigeminal neuralgia.

Pharmacological approaches

The World Health Organization (WHO) Analgesic Ladder, first published in 2006, recommends treating pain based on severity [4] (Figure 1.1). Mild pain should be treated with nonopioid analgesics (acetaminophen or nonsteroidal anti-inflammatory drugs), moderate pain should be treated with "weak" opioids, and severe pain should be treated with "strong" opioids. Adjuvants can be combined with analgesics for the treatment of pain of any severity, depending on the nature of pain (see Chapter 2). Although it was first proposed for the treatment of cancer-related pain, the WHO pain ladder was soon extrapolated to chronic nonmalignant pain.

Several authors have proposed modifications to the WHO pain ladder in recent years, due to developing scientific evidence. Eisenberg et al [5]

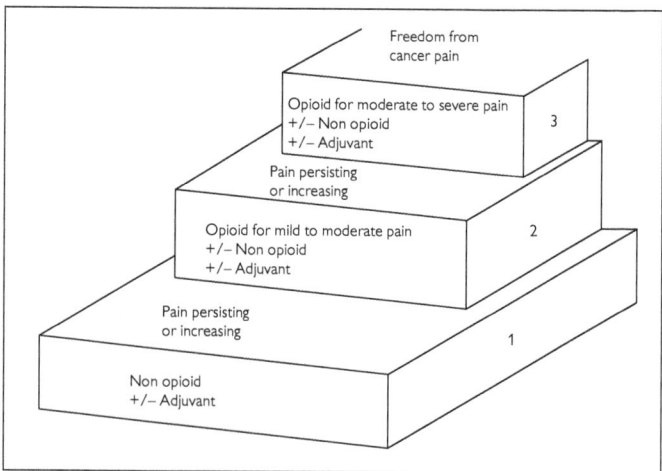

Figure 1.1 WHO analgesic ladder [4].

proposed to eliminate weak opioids for the treatment of cancer pain, because low doses of strong opioids have been shown to provide better and faster pain relief, with greater patient satisfaction [6]. Invasive procedures should be considered at any stage, as an alternative or an adjunct to pharmacotherapy.

Vargas-Schaffer [7] proposed to keep steps 1–3 unchanged and add a fourth step for managing the crises of chronic pain, comprising nerve block, epidurals, patient-controlled analgesia pump, neurolytic block therapy, and spinal stimulators. The treatment should also be adapted to the nature and acuteness of pain, using a "step up" approach for chronic pain, nonmalignant pain, and cancer pain and a "step down" approach for acute pain, chronic pain without control, and acute crises of chronic pain.

Although evidence is still limited, there is proof that pain is better controlled, with fewer adverse effects, when using a combination of diverse classes of analgesics [8] (see Chapter 4 for examples). It is clinical experience derived from clinical practice. Therefore, when clinicians select the most appropriate analgesics for a given patient, they should combine various analgesics with different mechanisms of action for a better pain relief.

Nonopioid analgesics

Acetaminophen is recommended as first-line therapy to treat mild to moderate pain, especially of musculoskeletal origin, because of the rarity of toxicity and adverse effects when used at therapeutic doses. Recent evidence and most guidelines recommend a maximal daily dose of 3200 mg when acetaminophen is used for more than 10 days in patients with risk factors for toxicity and 2600 mg in patients with other risk factors (polypharmacy, advanced age, alcohol abuse, liver impairment). When used to treat acute pain of less than 10-day duration, the traditional 4000 mg maximal daily dose can be used. When acetaminophen is administered on a chronic basis, frequent monitoring of liver function tests should be done to avoid liver toxicity.

Nonsteroidal anti-inflammatory drugs and selective cyclooxygenase-2 inhibitors are indicated for the treatment of inflammatory diseases (eg, rheumatoid arthritis) or for the treatment of acute pain. Nonsteroidal anti-inflammatory drugs are associated with significant adverse effects, including acute kidney injury, hyperkalemia, gastric toxicity, fluid retention, congestive heart failure, and possibly increased cardiac mortality; therefore, they should be used with caution, especially in older patients or those with several comorbidities or polypharmacy, with frequent monitoring for the occurrence of adverse effects.

Opioids

As indicated earlier, opioids should be used for the treatment of pain of moderate or severe intensity. Treatment should be initiated with a low dose and increased progressively based on analgesic response and tolerability. Responses to various opioids can vary depending on the patient and type of pain. Opioid rotation can be done when pain does not respond to a specific opioid. When prescribing an opioid, it is always important to first evaluate the risk of medication abuse and diversion and then frequently reassess these issues.

Conclusion

This chapter provides a very brief overview of pain management. To ensure optimal pain management, a combination of various pain relief strategies should be used, with a multimodal and interprofessional approach, combining nonpharmacological, pharmacological, interventional, and specific approaches. Pharmacotherapy should also include various classes of analgesics with different mechanisms of action, for better pain relief and tolerability.

References

1. Merskey H, Bogduk N, eds. *Classification of Chronic Pain, Second Edition*. Seattle, WA: IASP Press; 1994.
2. American Society of Anesthesiologists Task Force on Chronic Pain Management, American Society of Regional Anesthesia and Pain Medicine. Practice guidelines for chronic pain management: an updated report by the American Society of Anesthesiologists Task Force on Chronic Pain Management and the American Society of Regional Anesthesia and Pain Medicine. Anesthesiology 2010; 112:810–833.
3. Keefe FJ, Porter L, Somer T, et al. Psychosocial interventions for managing pain in older adults: outcomes and clinical implications. Br J Anaesth 2013; 111:89–94.
4. World Health Organization. WHO's pain ladder. Available at: www.who.int/cancer/palliative/painladder/en/. Accessed 9 September 2014.
5. Eisenberg E, Marinangeli F, Birkhahm J, et al. Time to modify the WHO analgesic ladder? Pain Clin Update 2005; 13:1–4.
6. Marinangeli F, Ciccozzi A, Leonardis M, et al. Use of strong opioids in advanced cancer pain: a randomized trial. J Pain Symptom Manage 2004; 27:409–416.
7. Vargas-Schaffer G. Is the WHO analgesic ladder still valid? Twenty-four years of experience. Can Fam Physician 2010; 56:514–517.
8. Chaparro LE, Wiffen PJ, Moore RA, Gilron I. Combination pharmacotherapy for the treatment of neuropathic pain in adults. Cochrane Database Syst Rev 2012; 7:CD008943.

Chapter 2

Classification of Analgesics

David Lussier and Pierre Beaulieu

Definition of adjuvant analgesics

The definition and concept of adjuvant analgesics have evolved considerably. In the initial World Health Organization (WHO) pain ladder [1], adjuvants were recommended "to calm fears and anxiety," that is, to treat accompanying symptoms, rather than as analgesics per se. The WHO later modified the definition of an adjuvant analgesic, distinguishing "coanalgesics" (anticonvulsants and antidepressants) and "adjuvant medicines" (steroids, muscle relaxants, and bisphophonates) [2]. This latter category corresponds to the accepted definition of an "adjuvant drug" as "a substance added to a drug to aid its action." After this definition was established, "adjuvants" were not considered as analgesics but were used to treat either a cause or contributing factor to pain; for example, steroids were used to treat inflammation and muscle relaxants were used to treat muscle spasms.

The definition and use of adjuvant analgesics have evolved with time. Nowadays, terms "adjuvant analgesic" and coanalgesic are often used interchangeably, and they have been defined as "any drug that has a primary indication other than pain, but is analgesic in some painful conditions" [3]. However, both adjuvant analgesic and coanalgesic terms have become obsolete with accumulating scientific evidence and evolution of prescription practices. Most drugs that are currently considered as adjuvant analgesics do not correspond to these definitions. They are often used alone rather than combined with an analgesic (eg, gabapentinoids or tricyclic antidepressants for neuropathic pain), and pain is an approved indication for some (eg, pregabalin, duloxetine).

This finding has lead some authors, including ourselves in a previous publication [4], to propose to completely abandon the terms and concept of adjuvant analgesics and simply consider them as analgesics if they have been shown to possess analgesic properties.

Existing classification of analgesics

Analgesics can be categorized based on different criteria, including severity of pain, type of pain, therapeutic classes of analgesics (eg, antidepressants, anticonvulsants), mechanisms of action, or a combination of different criteria. Several classifications have been proposed (Table 2.1).

Table 2.1 Categories of Classifications of Analgesics

Based on pain severity
WHO pain ladder [1]
Based on clinical efficacy
Lussier and Portenoy [3]
Based on therapeutic class
Based on pain mechanisms (mechanistic approaches)
Marchand [5]
Costigan and Woolf [6]
Lussier and Beaulieu [4]

World Health Organization classification

The first classification of analgesics, which remains classic, was presented by WHO for the treatment of cancer pain and was later extrapolated for noncancer pain (Table 2.2) [1]. In this classification, known as the WHO pain ladder, the treatment is based on pain severity. Nonopioid analgesics (acetaminophen or nonsteroidal anti-inflammatory drugs [NSAIDs]) are used for mild pain, whereas "weak" opioids (hydrocodone, codeine, low-dose oxycodone) are used for moderate pain and "strong" opioids (morphine, hydromorphone, high-dose oxycodone, fentanyl, methadone) are used for severe pain. Adjuvant drugs are recommended to calm fears and anxiety. A more recent but less known WHO classification categorizes analgesics as nonopioids, opioids, coanalgesics (antidepressants, anticonvulsants, ketamine, local anesthetics), or adjuvants (steroids, muscle relaxants, bisphosphonates) [2].

Table 2.2 World Health Organization Pain Ladder [1]

Analgesics for Mild Pain
Nonopioids
Acetaminophen
Nonsteroidal anti-inflammatory drugs (NSAIDs)
Analgesics for Moderate Pain
"Weak opioids"
Hydrocodone
Codeine
Low-dose oxycodone
Analgesics for Severe Pain
"Strong opioids"
Morphine
Hydromorphone
High-dose oxycodone
Fentanyl
Methadone
Adjuvant Analgesics

Classification based on clinical efficacy

The most commonly used and clinically relevant classification of adjuvant analgesics is based on clinical efficacy, for example, multipurpose, neuropathic pain, bone pain, and musculoskeletal pain [3] (Table 2.3). The pitfall of this type of classification is the evolving knowledge on analgesic efficacy of various drugs, which would require frequent modifications to the classification.

Classification based on therapeutic class

Adjuvant analgesics are then categorized based on their original therapeutic class and indication, for example, antidepressants, anticonvulsants, muscle relaxants, antiarrythmics. This categorization can often be misleading because it might imply that either all drugs from the class have analgesic properties or all drugs from the same class have similar mechanisms of action, neither of which is true. It can also be misleading to patients, who may believe they are prescribed an antidepressant to treat depression.

Classifications based on pain mechanisms

Rather than classifying analgesics based on their clinical efficacy or therapeutic class, these classifications, called "mechanistic approaches", divide analgesics

Table 2.3 Classification Based on Clinical Efficacy, From Lussier and Portenoy [3]

Multipurpose Adjuvant Analgesics
Antidepressants
Corticosteroids
α_2-Adrenergic agonists
Adjuvant Analgesics Used for Neuropathic Pain
First Line:
Gabapentinoid anticonvulsants
Antidepressants
Corticosteroids
Other drugs:
Oral and parenteral sodium channel blockers
N-methyl-D-aspartate (NMDA) receptor blockers
Cannabinoids
Baclofen
Adjuvant Analgesics Used for Bone Pain
Calcitonin and bisphosphonates
Radiopharmaceuticals
Corticosteroids
Adjuvant Analgesics Used for Bowel Obstruction
Anticholinergics
Octreotide
Corticosteroids
Adjuvant Analgesics Used for Musculoskeletal Pain

depending on which pain mechanism they act on or even on the molecular targets. According to Marchand [5], the most appropriate analgesic can then be determined based on the specific mechanism of the patient's pain, for example, nociceptive (somatic, visceral, inflammatory) or neuropathic (complex regional pain syndrome, peripheral and central neuropathic pain, spinal cord injury, functional pain) (Table 2.4).

In contrast to Marchand [5], Costigan and Woolf [6] have divided pain mechanisms into peripheral sensitization, ectopic discharge, sympathetically maintained pain, central sensitization, and reduced inhibition or increased transmission (Table 2.5). Moreover, each mechanism is further divided in various molecular targets of analgesics.

Finally, in a previous publication, we have proposed a taxonomy of analgesics inspired by previously existing classifications and based mainly on mechanisms of analgesia [4] (Table 2.6). It completely eliminates the term "adjuvant analgesic" and considers them as analgesics, on the same level as nonopioids and opioids. Investigational drugs can be easily added to the classification based on their mechanism of action, which should eliminate the need for frequent modifications to the taxonomy with evolving knowledge.

Table 2.4 Mechanistic Classification of Pain, From Marchand [5]

Type of Pain		Mechanisms	Example of Pharmacologic Treatments
Nociceptive	Somatic (tissue injury)	Mechanical, thermal, or chemical stimuli	Acetaminophen Sodium channel blockers NSAIDs Steroids Opioids
	Visceral (irritable bowel, cystitis)	Visceral distension	NSAIDs Antispasmodics
	Inflammatory (musculoskeletal)	Associated with localized inflammation	NSAIDs Steroids
Neurogenic	Causalgia (neuralgia, radiculopathy, CNS lesions)	Peripheral or CNS lesions	Anticonvulsants Opioids Antidepressants
	Functional (fibromyalgia, thalamic syndromes, irritable bowel)	Dysregulation of excitatory or inhibitory mechanisms in CNS	Antidepressants Anticonvulsants Opioids Cannabinoids

Abbreviations: CNS, central nervous system; NSAIDs, nonsteroidal anti-inflammatory drugs.

Table 2.5 Drug Treatment Based on Pain Mechanism Molecular Targets, From Costigan and Woolf [6]

Mechanism	Target	Drug
Peripheral sensitization	TRPV1	Capsaicin
Ectopic discharge	TTXs Na^+ -VGSC TTXr Na^+ -VGSC	Sodium channel blockers Carbamazepine Lamotrigine Mexiletine Lidocaine
Sympathetically maintained pain	α_1-receptor	Phentolamine Guanethidine block
Central sensitization	NMDA receptor	NMDA antagonists Ketamine
	COX-2	Dextromethorphan COX-2 selective inhibitors
Reduced inhibition Increased transmission	Receptors MOR, α_2, GABA, N-type Ca^{2+} channels	μ-opioid agonists, gabapentin, clonidine, tricyclic antidepressants

Abbreviations: α_1/α_2, adrenergic receptor subtypes; COX-2, cyclooxygenase subtype 2; GABA, γ-aminobutyric acid; MOR, μ-opioid receptor; NMDA, N-methyl-D-aspartate receptor; TRPV1, vanilloid receptor subtype 1; TTXr Na^+ -VGSC, tetrodotoxin-resistant-voltage-gated sodium channel; TTXs Na^+ -VGSC, tetrodotoxin-sensitive-voltage-gated sodium channel.

Table 2.6 Mechanistic Taxonomy of Analgesics, From Beaulieu and Lussier [4]

Antinociceptive Analgesics
Nonopioids
  Acetaminophen
  NSAIDs
Opioids
Cannabinoids

Antihyperalgesics
  NMDA antagonists
  Gabapentinoids (gabapentin, pregabalin)
  Levetiracetam
  Lamotrigine
  Nefopam
  Nitrous oxide
  Coxibs

Modulators of Descending Inhibition or Excitation
  Tricyclic Antidepressants
  SNRIs

(continued)

Table 2.6 Continued

SSRIs
α_2-adrenergic agonists
Modulators of Peripheral Transmission or Sensitization
Local anesthetics
Carbamazepine
Oxcarbazepine
Topiramate
Capsaicin
Mixed: Antinociceptive Analgesics and Modulators of Descending Inhibition or Excitation
Tramadol
Tapentadol
Other
Calcitonin
Bisphosphonates

Abbreviations: Coxibs, selective cyclooxygenase-2-inhibitors; NMDA, N-methyl-D-aspartate; NSAIDs, nonsteroidal anti-inflammatory drugs; SNRIs, serotonin-norepinephrine reuptake inhibitors; SSRIs, selective serotonin reuptake inhibitors.

References

1. World Health Organization. WHO's pain ladder. Available at: www.who.int/cancer/palliative/painladder/en/. Accessed 29 August 2014.

2. World Health Organization. Treatment guidelines on pain related to cancer, HIV and other progressive life-threatening illnesses in adults. Adopted in WHO Steering Group on Pain Guidelines, October 14, 2008. Available at: http://www.who.int/medicines/areas/quality_safety/Scoping_WHOGuide_non-malignant_pain_adults.pdf. Accessed 18 November, 2014.

3. Lussier D, Portenoy RK. Adjuvant analgesics in pain management. In: Hanks G, Cherny N, Christakis N, et al, eds. *Oxford Textbook of Palliative Medicine*, 4th edition. Oxford, England: Oxford University Press, 2010; pp. 707–734.

4. Lussier D, Beaulieu P. Toward a rational taxonomy of analgesics. In: Beaulieu P, Lussier D, Porreca F, Dickenson AH, eds. *Pharmacology of Pain*. Seattle, WA: IASP Press, 2010; pp. 27–40.

5. Marchand S. The physiology of pain mechanisms: from the periphery to the brain. Rheum Dis Clin North Am 2008; 34:285–309.

6. Costigan M, Woolf CJ. Pain: molecular mechanisms. J Pain 2000; 1(Suppl 1):35–44.

Chapter 3

Antidepressants

C. Peter N. Watson

> "I do believe," said Alice at last, "that they live in the same house!"
> LEWIS CARROLL, *Through the Looking Glass*

Introduction

The quotation refers to both the independent analgesic action and the dual action on inhibitory monoaminergic neurotransmitters of some antidepressants. Antidepressants are one of the oldest pharmacological treatments for chronic pain, and they have been subjected to many randomized controlled trials (RCTs) for chronic noncancer pain (CNCP) [1]. More than a quarter century of investigation has resulted in a large amount of literature on this topic. This chapter is based on systematic reviews of quality RCTs in chronic non-cancer pain [1–5]. Historically, these RCTs first examined tricyclic antidepressants (TCAs) such as amitriptyline based on published observational data and because of their putative action on potentiating pain-inhibitory mechanisms involving serotonin and noradrenaline. Because of limitations in efficacy and concern about adverse effects, attention turned to the more selective serotonin re-uptake inhibitors (SSRIs) such as fluoxetine and others and the more noradrenergic (N) agents such as maprotiline, desipramine, and nortriptyline. More recently, because of disappointing results regarding the superiority of most of these more specific antidepressants (except the more N TCA nortriptyline [6]), recent research has explored new drugs such as the serotonin noradrenaline re-uptake inhibitors (SNRIs) venlafaxine, duloxetine, and milnacipran, which, similar to amitriptyline, have an effect on both serotonin and noradrenaline with the hope of fewer adverse effects and better analgesia.

This chapter reviews (1) pharmacological aspects (dose, duration, pharmacodynamics, adverse effects) of these drugs (Table 3.1) and (2) the evidence-based data concerning clinical meaningfulness regarding efficacy and safety in CNCP (arthritis, fibromyalgia [FM], headache, low back pain, miscellaneous chronic pain, and particularly neuropathic pain [NP]) (Table 3.2). The TCAs, SSRIs, and combined SNRIs are considered here. There is evidence of an analgesic action of some of the antidepressants by RCTs and the relief of different components of NP in particular; that is, steady pain, jabbing, and evoked pain (allodynia). Other analgesics can now be regarded

Table 3.1 Analgesic Antidepressants (Dose, Duration, Pharmacodynamics, Adverse Effects)

Drug	Therapeutic Range for Pain (mg/24 h)	Half-life (h)	Neurotransmitter Profile		Most Common Side Effects (%)					
			NA	5-HT	Sedation	Orthostatic hypotension	Weight gain	Dry mouth	Constipation	GI distress, nausea, diarrhea
Tricyclics										
Amitriptyline	10–150*	10–46	+++	+++	>30	>10	>30	>30	>10	>2
Doxepin	10–150*	8–36	+++	++	>30	>10	>10	>30	>10	<2
Trimipramine	10–150*	7–30	++	+	>30	>10	>10	>10	>10	<2
Imipramine	10–150*	4–34	+++	+++	>10	>30	>10	>30	>10	>10
Clomipramine	10–150*	17–37	+++	++++	>2	>10	>10	>30	>10	>10
Desipramine	10–150*	12–76	+++++	++	>2	>2	>2	>10	>2	>2
Nortriptyline	10–100*	13–88	++++	++	>2	>2	>2	>10	>10	<2
Serotonin/Noradrenaline Reuptake Inhibitors										
Venlafaxine Effexor	37.5–225	3–7 (parent) 9–13 (metabolite)	++	++++	>10	>10	<2	>10	>10	>30
Duloxetine Cymbalta	60–120	10	++++	+++++	>10	<10	<2	>10	>10	>10

Abbreviations: GI, gastrointestinal; NA, not applicable; 5-HT, 5-hydroxytryptamine.

*The therapeutic range for depression is up to 200 mg/24 h for nortriptyline and to 300 mg/24 h for the remaining tricyclic antidepressants; in general, these doses are not required for an analgesic effect, and the usual dose will consist of 75 mg/24 h or less.

Adapted from Reference 5 with permission.

Table 3.2 Average NNT Among Placebo-Controlled Trials Examining TCAs, and Serotonin and Noradrenaline Reuptake Inhibitor Antidepressants for Neuropathic Pain for Benefit (50% or More Reduction of Pain), and Minor and Major Harm

Agent*	NNT "Benefit"	NNT "Minor Harm"	NNT "Major Harm"**	Number of Studies[+]
Amitriptyline	2.4	20.4	30.5	6
Imipramine	2.1	1.4	13.7	4
Desipramine	2.4	12.4	15.2	3
Nortriptyline	2.6	1.4	–	3
Clomipramine	2.1	No dichotomous data available	8.7	1
Average TCAs	2.3	8.9	17	
Venlafaxine	4.0			2
SSRIs	6.7			3

Abbreviations: NNT, numbers needed to treat; SSRIs, selective serotonin re-uptake inhibitors; TCA, tricyclic antidepressants.

*References for several sources of NNT figures are found in Reference 5.

**Major harm consists of withdrawal from the study due to adverse effects.

[+]This column refers to the number of studies for which there was adequate information with which to calculate an average NNT. Please note that these figures derive from studies using different methodologies, different data analyses, with different numbers of patients. There are few comparative trials, and the external validity may be poor because of selection that goes into trials. Thus, the NNT data are a rough guide only.

Adapted from Reference 5 with permission.

as first-line therapy (the gabapentinoids), but there is no good evidence for abandoning TCAs as an initial choice. Evidence is provided for the lesser utility of more selective serotonergic (S) and N agents and SNRIs [7]. There are few head-to-head RCTs [8], and comparative data are predominantly based on number-needed-to-treat (NNT) and number-needed-to-harm (NNH) figures [13] (Table 3.2). Evidence-based guidelines from different countries (Canada, United States, and Europe) [9–14] have reasonable concordance. The limited external validity (generalizability to ordinary practice) [15] of these drugs and the limited efficacies of drugs often lead to the need for combinations of antidepressants with anticonvulsants and opioids in many patients. Finally, we provide practical guidelines for the use of antidepressants in chronic pain.

Mechanism of action

Randomized controlled trials have repeatedly and clearly demonstrated the separation of the analgesic and antidepressant effects [16, 17]. An early concept of the mechanism of antidepressant analgesia was that this analgesia occurred via pain-inhibiting systems that descend from the brainstem on to the dorsal horn of the spinal cord [18]. This model involves an endorphin link from the periaqueductal gray area to the medullary raphe nucleus and then an S connection from the raphe to the dorsal horn of the spinal cord. However, another inhibitory system extends from the locus coeruleus in the lateral pons to the dorsal horn, which involves noradrenalin. More recently, descending facilitation by an S mechanism has been described [19]. This may explain the lesser or lack of efficacy of selective S drugs such as the SSRIs. Randomized controlled trials have demonstrated that the selective S drugs are either not effective [20] or less effective than N agents and those with a mixed effect on S and N (TCAs, SNRIs). The more effective antidepressants for chronic pain seem to be the TCAs desipramine, amitriptyline and its metabolite nortriptyline. Antidepressants are relatively "dirty drugs" that act on multiple receptors and have multiple effects (dopamine potentiation, the anticholinergic effect, an antihistaminic effect, an anti-inflammatory effect due to the inhibition of prostaglandin synthetase, an opioid-mediated effect, K^+ channel activation, $GABA_B$ potentiation, substance P reduction, or a calcium channel blocking action). Recent attractive ideas, in light of current thinking, are that these drugs may be *N*-methyl-D-aspartate antagonists or sodium channel blockers. In this chapter, we will focus on the monoamine descending inhibition model and use this model to categorize and explain the efficacy of the analgesic antidepressants. Aggressive pharmaceutical marketing of newer SNRI antidepressants for both NP and FM has created an impression among clinicians that those are the first-line pharmacotherapy for these indications; however, the evidence base does not support this assertion [7].

Acute and cancer pain

Use of antidepressants for acute and cancer pain is discussed in Chapters 9.4 and 9.2, respectively, as well as in Reference [1].

Neuropathic pain

The definition, assessment methods, and most common etiologies of NP are provided in Chapter 9.1. Most antidepressant research has been carried out in NP, and 80% of NP RCTs have been done in painful diabetic neuropathy (PDN) and postherpetic neuralgia (PHN). Sixty-one RCTs of 20 antidepressants in NP were identified [1]. Seventeen were conducted in PDN, 11 in PHN, and 33 in other NP conditions, which included facial pain, NP with cancer, central poststroke pain, human immunodeficiency virus (HIV) neuropathy, spinal cord injury, cisplatin neuropathy, painful polyneuropathy, phantom limb pain, and chronic lumbar root pain. Of the trials of oral drugs, 13 antidepressants in 36 RCTs showed a significant effect. With TCAs, six drugs tested favorably, including amitriptyline, imipramine, nortriptyline, desipramine, and nortriptyline. Of SNRIs, venlafaxine and duloxetine were superior to placebo. Selective serotonin re-uptake inhibitors yielded favorable results over placebo with paroxetine, citalopram, and escitalopram. The tetracyclic, N maprotiline (3 RCTs), and the N/dopaminergic bupropion (one RCT) also have shown a significant effect compared with placebo. These RCTs have repeatedly shown an analgesic effect independent of an effect on depression and the relief of the different pain qualities seen in NP, including steady pain, jabbing pain, and skin pain (allodynia or pain on touch). Randomized controlled trials results in

PDN and PHN are reasonably similar, but negative trials in such NP disorders as lumbar root pain, HIV and cisplatin neuropathies, and spinal cord injury may reflect the greater intractability of these NP problems.

A significant difficulty for the clinician lies in interpreting the results of these many RCTs for translation to clinical practice in deciding which drug to use. One problem is the lack of clinical meaningfulness data in most studies such as the number of subjects with satisfactory relief [15]. Another issue is the paucity of comparative data (most RCTs are a comparison with placebo) [8]. To address these deficiencies, NNT figures for 50% or more relief and NNH figures for withdrawal for NP RCTs have been calculated for both antidepressants and other analgesic classes [13] (Table 3.2). In NP, these data indicate that balanced N/S TCAs are superior to N TCAs and SNRIs, which in turn are superior to SSRIs. In addition, TCA NNTs are about equal to the opioids morphine and oxycodone and superior to gabapentinoids (gabapentin, pregabalin), the opioid-like drug tramadol, and cannabinoids. These data are helpful in placing the different drugs in a treatment algorithm for NP [9], which places TCAs as a first choice along with gabapentinoids and SNRIs as a second choice.

Fibromyalgia

A systematic review of the effectiveness of antidepressants in FM in 2008 [21] was based on 26 RCTs. The authors concluded that amitriptyline (10–50 mg/day) reduced pain, fatigue, and depression in FM and improved sleep and quality of life. They also found that some SSRIs and the SNRIs duloxetine and milnacipran were effective but that long-term data were lacking.

A meta-analysis [22] of 18 RCTs of antidepressants concluded that antidepressants were associated with improvements in pain, depression, fatigue, sleep, and health-related quality of life in patients with FM. Results of the analysis also indicated large effect sizes for TCAs (mostly amitriptyline), a medium effect size for monoamine oxidase (MAO) inhibitors (moclobemide, pirlindole), and a small effect size for SSRIs (fluoxetine, citalopram, paroxetine) and SNRIs (duloxetine, milnacipran).

The literature review for this chapter [1] found further favorable results for three trials of the SNRIs duloxetine (20–120 mg/day) and four RCTs of milnacipran. As a class of drugs, dual uptake inhibitors improved pain, depression, sleep, and quality of life in several of these studies.

Headache

Four antidepressants were favorable in 16 RCTs in tension-type headache, migraine, and medication-induced and chronic daily headache [1, 4]. Of the commercially available drugs, those with a mixed effect on serotonin and noradrenaline (ie, amitriptyline, venlafaxine, and mirtazapine) were superior in both migraine and tension headache, but amitriptyline was superior in only one RCT in drug withdrawal headache. The SSRIs were found to be no more effective than placebo in migraine and less effective than TCAs in chronic tension-type headaches [1, 4]. Thus, the TCA amitriptyline, the tetracyclic mirtazapine, and the SNRI venlafaxine all seem useful for headache prevention of both migraine and tension-type headaches. Most RCTs report a reduction in duration and frequency of headache and, less commonly, of severity.

Low back pain

Three antidepressants were favorable for low back pain (amitriptyline, nortriptyline, and doxepin) [1, 3].

Arthritis

Amitriptyline, imipramine, and trimipramine were found to be favorable for different arthritis conditions (osteoarthritis, rheumatoid arthritis, ankylosing spondylitis) [1].

Adverse events

Table 3.1 summarizes monoamine profiles and common side effects for some commonly used antidepressants, and more details are available elsewhere [1, 23]. If insomnia accompanies pain, a sedating TCA may be chosen (such as amitriptyline) and given in a single nightime dose, which may also mitigate unwanted daytime drowsiness. The presence of a seizure disorder precludes the use of bupropion. Allergic reactions are generally uncommon. Withdrawal reactions may occur and gradual withdrawal is prudent. Number-needed-to-harm figures for TCAs do not indicate a worse side-effect profile in RCTs than other drug choices for CNCP such as gabapentinoids (Table 3.2) [13]. Most SNRIs are unlikely to cause severe anticholinergic, adrenergic, and antihistaminic side effects, severe sedation, hypotension, and weight gain. They may cause gastrointestinal upset (commonest), insomnia, dry mouth, drowsiness, sweating, anxiety, agitation, headache, sexual dysfunction, and tremor. A central S syndrome and an increased risk of gastrointestinal bleeding have been reported. Serotonin norepinephrine re-uptake inhibitors may aggravate hypertension, exacerbate seizures, and trigger mania. More common are nausea, anorexia, weakness, drowsiness, nervousness, dizziness, and dry mouth. Drug interactions are a consideration with all antidepressants, and the safety of most antidepressants in pregnancy and lactation has not been established.

Drug Selection

There are numerous largely placebo-controlled RCTs in CNCP, indicating that a variety of antidepressants are superior to placebo in many conditions. These trials may leave the clinician in a state of confusion as to the appropriate choice of agent because there are few head-to-head comparative trials and sparse data on the clinical meaningfulness of results in individual RCTs in terms of the number of subjects obtaining satisfactory relief. The few head-to-head RCTs most commonly indicate the superiority of nonselective TCA antidepressants over SNRIs and SSRIs [8]. To further judge the relative efficacy and safety of these drugs in comparison with each other and with other analgesics such as gabapentinoids and opioids, NNTs for 50% or more relief and NNHs for RCT withdrawal have been calculated in NP where there are substantial numbers of RCTs [5] (Table 2). This helps to rank these drugs in terms of NNT values in RCTs in NP trials as balanced S/N TCAs > N antidepressants > SNRIs > SSRIs. For comparison with other analgesics, NNT values for gabapentinoids are 5.1 for gabapentin, 4.2 for pregabalin, 2.5 for opioids (morphine, oxycodone), and 4 for the dual mechanism agent tramadol. Number-needed-to-harm figures for withdrawal from RCTs for TCAs are 14.7, 26.2 for gabapentin, and 11.7 for pregabalin. Treatment algorithms suggested for NP often recommend a TCA such as amitriptyline or nortriptyline or a gabapentinoid (gabapentin, pregabalin) as first choice (depending on age, concomitant disorders, and side effects) and an SNRI (venlafaxine, duloxetine) as second choice. Due to lack of sufficient evidence, other antidepressants are recommended for NP refractory to other therapies (see Chapter 9.1).

In FM, effect size data suggest that TCAs (amitriptyline) are superior to the medium effect size of the MAO inhibitors (moclobemide, pirlindole) and the small effect size of the SSRIs and SNRIs (duloxetine, milnacipran) studied [21]. Of commercially available drugs for migraine and tension headaches, balanced drugs such as the TCA amitriptyline, the SNRI venlafaxine, and the tetracyclic mirtazapine may be useful prophylactically. For chronic low back pain, arthritis, and the miscellaneous CNCP group, general guidelines such as those for NP seem reasonable because there are few studies.

An important issue is the generalizability (external validity) of data from RCTs where patients are usually selected according to many inclusion and exclusion criteria [15]. Most of the antidepressant research in NP has been carried out in PHN and PDN, which have proven to be good clinical experimental models, but it is unclear whether this model can be applied to other NP or other causes of CNCP. An RCT NNT result of 2 or 3 will almost certainly not be achieved in ordinary practice where patients are older, are on other drugs, and have other disorders. The results of all analgesics in RCTs in CNCP indicate a moderate effect at best in the selected subjects chosen. Currently, for antidepressants, it seems that either we have not struck the right balance of serotonin and noradrenaline or that descending monoamine systems are only one component of pain inhibition. Combinations of drugs may be necessary (tricyclics, gabapentinoids, opioids, cannabinoids) unless a "magic bullet" is found, but this solution does not seem to be imminent.

Approach to therapy

In selecting an antidepressant such as a TCA for CNCP, it is important to (1) individualize therapy, (2) obtain a complete assessment, and (3) focus on issues that may preclude these drugs such as advanced age, heart disease (recent myocardial infarction, conduction defects), urinary retention, glaucoma, other medications, and alcohol intake. In deciding on antidepressant therapy, a history of failed antidepressant usage should not dissuade one from a careful trial because many failures result from high initial dosing, noncompliance, or an inadequate trial (too low a dose or too brief a trial). It is important to carefully explain the goals of treatment and adverse effects to patients. They need to understand that complete relief is possible but unlikely and that the aim of treatment is to take the pain from severe or moderate to mild (occurs in 50%–60% in RCTs). Patients also need to know that the starting dose will be low and will be slowly increased (every week or so) until satisfactory relief occurs or an intolerable adverse effect is experienced. It is important to inform them that the effect of a dose increase may not be experienced for one week or more and that, if stopped, side effects are probable (the most common with TCAs being dry mouth, constipation, and drowsiness) and that, if stopped, drug withdrawal should be gradual. A sedating TCA (amitriptyline) may be useful with the total dose at bedtime if insomnia is a problem or to avoid daytime drug-induced drowsiness. Weight gain may occur with some agents, in which case diet and appropriate weight monitoring are important, particularly in the already overweight population. Sexual dysfunction may be more important in the younger age groups. Less common adverse effects are allergic reactions such as rash, tachycardia (usually supraventricular), and paradoxical insomnia. If possible, it is prudent to eliminate all other ineffective analgesics and sedating drugs so that drug interactions (such as sedation and constipation) are minimized. Antidepressants may interact with other non-analgesics such as those that either prolong the QT interval (eg, methadone) or interfere with hepatic metabolism (via cytochrome P450), possibly causing ventricular tachycardia (antiarrythmics, antiretrovirals, antifungals, calcium channel blockers, macrolide and quinolone antibiotics, SSRIs, antipsychotics, tamoxifen, and cisapride) (see Chapter 10).

Useful baseline tests are blood pressure measurement supine and standing, hematology, liver and kidney function, electrolytes, and an electrocardiogram. A good general principle is to "start low and go slow," keeping in mind that with TCAs the analgesic effect occurs at lower doses than the antidepressant effect (mean, 50–75 mg). If treatment is started with a TCA such as nortriptyline (less significant adverse events) or amitriptyline, it is reasonable to begin with 10 mg for patients over 65 and 25 mg for those under 65 and then slowly increase the dose every week or two by similar amounts until an end point of satisfactory pain relief or a significant adverse event. It may be helpful to try different antidepressants and move from TCAs (nortriptyline, amitriptyline, desipramine, imipramine) to the SNRIs (venlafaxine and duloxetine) because individual differences in pain inhibitory mechanisms may mean that one drug is more efficacious for an individual patient. In addition, close follow-up (every 2 weeks initially) is important to supervise compliance, dose increments, and to deal with adverse effects. Preemptive prescription of a stool softener and an artificial saliva mouth spray are useful routine measures. There is no therapeutic range of blood levels for antidepressants, but they can be useful to check compliance and as a guide to dose increments in some patients who require higher doses. In some patients, good relief and therapeutic blood levels may be achieved with low doses of 10–20 mg, but it is important to note that this response may not always be age-related. A three-month treatment trial is reasonable; combination therapy is reasonable and necessary in refractory cases (gabapentinoids, opioids, cannabinoids, topical agents).

In CNCP, head-to-head RCTs, NNT figures, and effect size data generally indicate the superiority of the TCAs (amitriptyline, nortriptyline, imipramine, desipramine) and a lesser effect of the SNRIs (venlafaxine, duloxetine, milnacipran) and SSRIs.

Summary

This chapter provides information about the pharmacology of antidepressants, guidelines and data regarding efficacy and safety from recent systematic reviews concerning antidepressants and pain and individual quality RCTs. Of particular interest in these studies are the clinical meaningfulness of the results and how the drugs compare with the standard therapy of the more specific subclass of TCAs and other analgesics. An important concern is the limited external validity or generalizability of trial data to the same disorders in ordinary practice. There are few head-to-head RCTs that compare different antidepressants with other analgesics. Indirect comparative measures such as NNT and NNH values are a useful additional means of comparison. Despite the increase in placebo-controlled RCTs of antidepressants in painful conditions, there has been no striking advance or "magic bullet" for monotherapy. There continues to be a need for comparative effectiveness research of new antidepressants by quality head-to-head RCTs comparing new drugs with old drugs to guide the clinician. Because of deficiencies in this area and because of evidence for poor generalizability, combinations of the useful antidepressants with other analgesic drugs need to be considered for many patients.

References

1. Watson CPN, Gilron I, Pollock BG, Lipman AG, Smith MT. Antidepressant analgesics. In: McMahon JR, Koltzenburg M, Tracey I, and Turck DC (eds.) *Wall and Melzack's Textbook of Pain*, 6th ed. Elsevier/Churchill Livingstone; 2012: pp. 465–490.

2. Saarto T, Wiffen PJ. Antidepressants in neuropathic pain (Review). The Cochrane Collaboration. The Cochrane Library: John Wiley & Sons Ltd. Available at: http://onlinelibrary.wiley.com/doi/10.1002/14651858.CD005454.pub2/abstract. 2007. Accessed 19 November, 2014.

3. Urquhart DM, Hoving JL, Assendelft WJ, et al. Antidepressants for non-specific low back pain (Review). The Cochrane Collaboration. The Cochrane Library: John Wiley & Sons, Ltd. Available at: http://onlinelibrary.wiley.com/doi/10.1002/14651858.CD001703.pub3/abstract. 2008.

4. Moja L, Cusi C, Sterzi R, et al. Selective serotonin re-uptake inhibitors for preventing migraine and tension headaches (Review). The Cochrane Collaboration. The Cochrane Library: John Wiley & Sons Ltd. Available

at: http://onlinelibrary.wiley.com/doi/10.1002/14651858.CD002919. pub2/abstract. 2005. Accessed 19 November, 2014.

5. Lynch ME, Watson CP. The pharmacotherapy of chronic pain: a review. Pain Res Manag 2006; 11:11–38.

6. Watson CP, Vernich L, Chipman M, Reed K. Nortriptyline versus amitriptyline in postherpetic neuralgia: a randomized trial. Neurology 1998; 51:1166–1171.

7. Watson CP, Gilron I, Sawynok J, Lynch ME. Nontricyclic antidepressants and pain: are the serotonin norepinephrine reuptake inhibitors any better? Pain 2011; 152:2206–2210.

8. Watson CP, Gilron I, Sawynok J. A qualitative, systematic review of head-to-head randomized, controlled trials of oral analgesics in neuropathic pain. J Pain Res Manag 2010; 15:147–157.

9. Moulin DE, Clark AJ, Gilron I, et al. Pharmacological management of chronic neuropathic pain-consensus statement and guidelines from the Canadian pain Society. Pain Res Manag 2007; 12:13–21.

10. Dworkin RH, O'Connor AB, Backonja M, et al. Pharmacologic management of neuropathic pain: evidence-based recommendations. Pain 2007; 132:237–251.

11. Attal N, Cruccu G, Baron R, et al. EFNS guidelines on the pharmacological treatment of neuropathic pain: 2010 revision. Eur J Neur 2010; 17:1113–1123.

12. O'Connor AB, Dworkin RH. Treatment of neuropathic pain: an overview of recent guidelines. Am J Med 2009; 122(10 Suppl):S22–S32.

13. Finnerup NB, Sindrup SH, Jensen TS. The evidence for pharmacological treatment of neuropathic pain. Pain 2010; 150:573–581.

14. Dworkin RH, O'Connor AB, Audette J, et al. Recommendations for the pharmacological management of neuropathic pain: an overview and literature update. Mayo Clin Proc 2010; 85(3 Suppl):S3–S14.

15. Watson CP. External validity of pharmaceutical trials in neuropathic pain. In: Rothwell PM, ed. *Treating Individuals: From Randomized Trials to Personalized Medicine*. Philadelphia: Elsevier; 2007: pp. 121–130.

16. Watson CP, Evans RJ, Reed K, et al. Amitriptyline versus placebo in postherpetic neuralgia. Neurology 1982; 32:671–673.

17. Max MB, Culnane M, Schafter SC, et al. Amitriptyline relieves diabetic neuropathy pain in patients with normal or depressed mood. Neurology 1987; 37:589–596.

18. Basbaum AI, Fields HL. Endogenous pain control mechanisms: review and hypothesis. Ann Neurol 1979; 4:451–462.

19. Bennarroch EE. Descending monoaminergic pain modulation. Neurology 2008; 71:217–221.

20. Max MB, Lynch SA, Muir J, et al. Effects of desipramine, amitriptyline, and fluoxetine on pain in diabetic neuropathy. N Engl J Med 1992; 326:1250–1256.

21. Uceyler N, Hauser W, Sommer C. A systematic review of the effectiveness of treatment with antidepressants in fibromyalgia syndrome. Arthritis Rheum 2008; 59:1279–1298.

22. Hauser W, Bernardy K, Uceyler N, et al. Treatment of fibromyalgia syndrome with antidepressants: a meta-analysis. JAMA 2009; 301:198–209.

23. Brunton L, Chabner B, Knollman B (eds) *Goodman and Gilman's Pharmacological Basis of Therapeutics*. 12th ed. New York: McGraw Hill; 2010.

Chapter 4

Anticonvulsants

David Lussier

Introduction

Several anticonvulsants have been shown to possess analgesic efficacy to various degrees and for different diseases. Historically, carbamazepine was used as early as 1962 for the treatment of trigeminal neuralgia. However, the gabapentinoids gabapentin and pregabalin are anticonvulsants that have been the most studied for analgesic activity, and they have been shown to be effective for neuropathic pain as well as for fibromyalgia. Other anticonvulsants have very limited evidence of analgesic efficacy, and they are only limited to neuropathic pain.

Mechanisms of action

The analgesic activity of most anticonvulsants results from a combination of diverse actions on the central nervous system, all decreasing central sensitization. These include sodium channel blockade, calcium channel blockade, suppression of glutamate release, and action on N-methyl-D-aspartate (NMDA) receptors [1].

Gabapentinoids

Gabapentin and pregabalin are thought to exert their analgesic action mostly via modulation of the $\alpha_2\delta$-1 protein of the N-type calcium channel. Gabapentin also acts on NMDA receptors, protein kinase C, and inflammatory cytokines [2]. A recent placebo-controlled study suggests that pregabalin reduces insular glutamatergic activity, which reduces the increased functional connectivity seen in chronic pain; neuroimaging markers predict analgesic response to pregabalin [3].

Gabapentin and pregabalin are both minimally bound to proteins and are not metabolized by the liver, and they are thereby devoid of pharmacokinetic drug-drug interactions. Pregabalin possesses a significant advantage over gabapentin, because it does not require active transporters to be absorbed, and therefore it has linear pharmacokinetics, which makes dose titration easier and allows twice-daily dosing [4]. Gabapentin, the saturable absorption process of which makes its bioavailability lower at higher doses (35% for 1600 mg three times daily vs 60% for a single 300 mg dose), requires administration 3–4 times daily [4]. However, the newer formulations of gastroretentive gabapentin and gabapentin enacarbil allows a once- and twice-daily administration, respectively. Pregabalin has a faster onset of action than gabapentin [5].

Gabapentin greatly expanded the use of anticonvulsants in pain management, due to several studies supporting its efficacy and its better tolerability than older anticonvulsants. Similarly to antidepressants, diabetic neuropathy [6, 7] and postherpetic neuralgia [8, 9] are the neuropathic conditions for which the analgesic efficacy of gabapentin has been the most studied, with several randomized controlled trials (RCTs) supporting it. Its use in acute herpes zoster [10], spinal cord injury [11], postthoracotomy pain [12], and lumbar spinal stenosis [13] is also supported by at least one RCT. Although limited to open-label trials, evidence also suggests it might be effective to treat pain from complex regional pain syndrome [14], human immunodeficiency virus (HIV) neuropathy [15], and multiple sclerosis [16], as well as cancer-related neuropathic pain (see Chapter 9.2). As explained in Chapter 9.1, comparative trials of analgesics of different classes for the management of neuropathic pain are very rare. When compared with amitriptyline, gabapentin was shown to be either equally [17] or more effective [7] and better tolerated [7] to treat diabetic neuropathy, whereas it was equally effective but better tolerated than nortriptyline to treat postherpetic neuralgia [18]. Albeit limited, there is some evidence that gabapentin might relieve pain from fibromyalgia [19].

Two new formulations of gabapentin have recently been introduced but are not yet marketed in all countries. A gastroretentive formulation, the pharmacokinetic properties of which allow daily administration of a 1800 mg dose, seems equally effective at similar doses, is better tolerated. and has a shorter titration period than immediate-release gabapentin [20], with efficacy and safety assessed for up to 24-week treatment [21]. Gabapentin enacarbil is an actively transported prodrug of gabapentin that provides sustained, dose-proportional exposure to gabapentin, allowing a twice-daily administration. Relief of pain associated with postherpetic neuralgia seems to occur at doses similar to gabapentin [22]. Evidence is supporting recommendation to use gastroretentive gabapentin as first-line therapy for postherpetic neuralgia, but it is still insufficient for gabapentin enacarbil [23].

Pregabalin, which possesses the same mechanism of action as gabapentin with better pharmacokinetic properties, has also been extensively studied and shown effective for diverse types of neuropathic pain, including painful diabetic neuropathy [24, 25] and postherpetic neuralgia [5]. Similarly to gabapentin, pregabalin was shown effective to treat central pain from spinal cord injury [26]. More importantly, prolonged 15-month benefits have been shown for neuropathic pain refractory to other adjuvant (gabapentin, antidepressants) and opioid analgesics [27]. In a meta-analysis of 17 RCTs evaluating 17 oral medications for chronic peripheral neuropathic pain and comprising close to 6000 subjects, 600 mg/day pregabalin had the largest beneficial effects along with 60 or 120 mg/day duloxetine [28]. Scientific data of its efficacy in fibromyalgia is sufficient to make it a first-line recommended analgesic (see Chapter 9.3). It can also relieve pain from irritable bowel syndrome and has been used for chronic pancreatitis [29]. Compared with a twice-daily administration of 300 mg, a single

300-mg night dose exerts similar analgesic effect in fibromyalgia-related pain, with reduced total adverse effects, however not specific to a particular adverse effect [30]. This supports clinical experience that a nightly administration is equally effective and better tolerated than a twice-daily dosing.

In one of the very few trials comparing analgesic efficacy of gabapentin and pregabalin, results showed that they were equally effective in treating painful peripheral neuropathy in hemodialysis patients, when given after each hemodialysis session, at doses of 300 and 75 mg, respectively [31]. Numbers needed to treat for gabapentin and pregabalin, compared with various antidepressants in neuropathic pain, are provided in Chapter 3.

There is accumulating evidence supporting a potential role for gabapentinoids in the perioperative period, to decrease either postoperative acute pain or opioid requirements (see Chapter 9.4). Perioperative administration of gabapentinoids might also reduce chronic postsurgical pain. Concomitant administration of 75 mg of pregabalin and 100 mg of celecoxib twice daily, started 14 days prior to a total hip arthroplasty and continued up to 3 weeks after hospital discharge, reduced movement-evoked pain and improved physical function [32]. However, according to a recent Cochrane meta-analysis of 10 and five RCTs of gabapentin and pregabalin, respectively, their administration before, during, or after surgery, or both, does not reduce the incidence of chronic pain 3 months after surgery [33].

Adverse effects, which are very similar for both drugs, are detailed in Table 4.1. Although uncommon, serious adverse effects have been reported, mostly neuropsychiatric, as well as hepatitis associated with gabapentin and hematological adverse effects associated with pregabalin [34]. Lethal adverse effects have been reported in obstetrical situations, which warrants caution in this patient population [34].

According to a recent Cochrane Database Review, only pregabalin and gabapentin have sufficient good quality evidence of an analgesic efficacy in neuropathic pain, using painful diabetic neuropathy and postherpetic neuralgia as models of neuropathic pain [35].

Carbamazepine and oxcarbazepine

Carbamazepine is still recommended as first-line therapy for trigeminal neuralgia, mostly for historical reasons [36] and based on old studies that suggested efficacy in trigeminal neuralgia (only for lancinating rather than continuous pain) [37] but also for painful diabetic neuropathy [38]. However, due to frequent adverse effects, including some potentially lethal such as leukopenia and Steven-Johnson syndrome, carbamazepine is very rarely used.

Oxcarbazepine, a metabolite of carbamazepine that was predicted to possess similar analgesic efficacy with better tolerability, did indeed show some effect in painful diabetic neuropathy [39] and postherpetic neuralgia [40], including in patients refractory to gabapentin [40]. However, other clinical trials in painful diabetic neuropathy and radiculopathy have failed to illustrate any benefit [41]. Furthermore, although most adverse effects are mild to moderate, serious adverse effects are not uncommon [41] (Table 4.1).

CHAPTER 4 Anticonvulsants

Table 4.1 Mechanism of action, dosing recommandations, contraindications and adverse effects of anticonvulsants most commonly used for pain management

Drug	Mechanism of Action	Starting Dose	Usual Effective dose	Precautions and Contraindications[1]	Commonly Reported Adverse Effects
Gabapentin immediate-release	Modulation of the alpha-2-delta-1 protein of the N-type calcium channel, which decreases central sensitization	100–300 mg daily; titrate by 100–300 mg every one to three days to an effective dose	300–1200 mg tid	Decrease dose in patients with renal dysfunction (avoid in severe renal dysfunction). Rapid discontinuation may result in headache, nausea, insomnia, and diarrhea.	Sedation, dizziness, tremor, peripheral oedema, weight gain, nausea, headache
Gastroretentive gabapentin		300 mg qd, titrate up to 1800 mg qd over 15 days	1800 mg qd		
Gabapentin enacarbil		600 mg qd, titrate to 600 mg bid after 3 days	600 mg bid		
Pregabalin		25–75 mg qd	150–300 mg bid[1]		
Carbamazepine	Blockage of voltage-gated sodium channels → ↓ cell excitability	100–200 mg qd-bid	300–800 mg bid	• Contraindicated in bone marrow depression, or within 14 days of MAOI use. • Caution in patients with cardiac disease, hepatic or renal dysfunction. • Potentially fatal blood dyscrasias have been reported; monitor CBC, platelets, renal and liver function, and serum sodium. • Potentially fatal severe dermatologic reactions (eg Stevens-Johnson syndromes) are rare.	Somnolence, dizziness, blurred vision, headache, confusion, speech and memory difficulties, cardiovascular abnormalities (eg arrhythmia, bradycardia, hypertension, AV block), rash, SIADH, nausea, urinary retention, hematologic abnormalities (eg aplastic anemia, bone marrow suppression, thrombocytopenia), increased liver enzymes, hepatic failure

Oxcarbazepine[2]	Idem as carbamazepine	150 mg qd; titrate by 150–300 mg every 3–5 days to an effective dose	150–600 mg bid	Clinically significant hyponatremia can develop: monitor serum sodium at baseline, during the first 3 months and periodically	Dizziness
Lamotrigine	1) Blockage of voltage-gated sodium channels → ↓ cell excitability 2) ↓ glutamatergic neurotransmission via glutamate receptors 3) ↑ GABAergic neurotrasmission	25 mg qd; titrate by 25 mg every 7 days to an effective dose	100–200 mg bid	Black box warning: severe and potentially life threatening skin rashes have been reported	Headache, dizziness, ataxia, somnolence, tremor, nausea, diarrhea, blurred vision, insomnia
Topiramate	1) Blockage of voltage-gated sodium channels → ↓ cell excitability 2) ↑ GABAergic neurotransmission	25–50 mg qd; titrate by 25 mg every 5–7 days to an effective dose	100–400 mg bid	• May significantly decrease serum bicarbonate; monitor serum bicarbonate at baseline and periodically. • Often poorly tolerated: high rate of withdrawal due to adverse effects	Somnolence, dizziness, ataxia, psychomotor slowing, speech and memory difficulties, decreased serum bicarbonate, metabolic acidosis, nausea, paresthesia, tremor, abnormal vision, nystagmus, diplopia, weight loss, nephrolithiasis, secondary angle closure glaucoma

(continued)

Table 4.1 Continued

Levetiracetam		250–500 mg bid	500–1500 mg bid		Somnolence, dizziness
Lacosamide	Unknown. Possible blockade of voltage-gated sodium channel	50 mg bid	200–400 mg bid		Dizziness, fatigue, nausea/vomiting
Zonisamide		100 mg qd	100–300 mg bid	• Use in patients with severe sulfonamide allergy is contraindicated; potentially fatal sulfonamide reactions (including Stevens-Johnson syndrome and toxic epidermal necrolysis) are rare. • Use cautiously in patients with renal or hepatic dysfunction.	Somnolence, dizziness, headache, confusion, ataxia, insomnia, tremor, nausea, weight loss, diplopia, nystagmus

[1] Pregabalin is better tolerated, and equally effective, with a single nightly dose rather than twice-daily dosing.

[2] ketoanalogue metabolite of carbamazepine.

Lamotrigine

Although analgesic efficacy of lamotrigine has been suggested for trigeminal neuralgia, HIV neuropathy, and central poststroke pain, studies on painful diabetic neuropathy have yielded conflicting results, and the addition of lamotrigine to either a nonopioid analgesic, gabapentin, or a tricyclic antidepressant did not provide further relief. Based on meta-analysis of this study, a recent Cochrane database review concluded that lamotrigine does not have a significant place in therapy for chronic neuropathic pain and fibromyalgia, especially given adverse effects of concern [42].

Topiramate

Individual randomized trials have shown that topiramate can relieve pain from diabetic neuropathy [43], chronic low back pain [44], and chronic lumbar radicular pain [45], as well as improve anger, subjective disability, and health-related quality of life in patients with low back pain [44]. Its analgesic effect might be exerted via decreased peripheral nerve excitability [46]. However, available evidence has been deemed insufficient to support its use in neuropathic pain [47].

Levetiracetam

Levetiracetam, which was once a promising agent due to animal and experimental data, good tolerability, and ease of dosing, has failed to show any analgesic efficacy in several pain conditions, including central neuropathic post-stroke pain [48], multiple sclerosis [49], and polyneuropathy [50].

Lacosamide

Lacosamide has been shown to be effective to treat neuropathic pain from diabetic neuropathy, but with a very mild effect, and it has failed to show benefits in fibromyalgia [51].

Zonisamide

Evidence for zonisamide is limited to one RCT in diabetic neuropathy [52].

Tiagabine

Evidence of analgesic efficacy for tiagabine is either anecdotal or limited to open-label studies.

Felbamate

Evidence of analgesic efficacy for felbamate is also either anecdotal or limited to open-label studies.

Because of very limited evidence of analgesic efficacy, lacosamide, zonisamide, tiagabine, and felbamate should only be considered as analgesics after trials of other analgesics with better evidence of efficacy.

Phenytoin, valproate, clonazepam

Despite large clinical experience and use, mostly before newer anticonvulsants were available, there is no good quality evidence on the analgesic activity of any of these drugs [35].

Conclusions

Anticonvulsants possess analgesic efficacy in a variety of painful conditions. Evidence is best for neuropathic pain, for which pregabalin, gabapentin, oxcarbazepine, lamotrigine, and topiramate have been shown to be effective, with much better evidence for the gabapentinoids. The latter also seem to possess some analgesic efficacy for fibromyalgia and the management of perioperative pain, including prevention of chronic postsurgical pain. With all medications, one should always consider potential benefits, common and serious adverse effects, as well as contraindications when considering prescribing an anticonvulsant as part of pharmacological management of pain, and clinicians should favor those with the best efficacy/adverse effects ratio.

References

1. Gilron I. The role of anticonvulsant drugs in postoperative pain management: a bench-to-bedside perspective. Can J Anesth 2006; 53:562–571.
2. Kukkar A, Bali A, Singh N, Jaggi AS. Implications and mechanism of action of gabapentin in neuropathic pain. Arch Pharm Res 2013; 36:237–251.
3. Harris RE, Napadow V, Huggins JP, et al. Pregabalin rectifies aberrant brain chemistry, connectivity, and functional response in chronic pain patients. Anesthesiol 2013; 119:1453–1464.
4. Perucca E. The clinical pharmacokinetics of the new antiepileptic drugs. Epilepsia 1999; 40 (Suppl 9):S7–S13.
5. Sabatowski R, Gálvez R, Cherry DA, et al. Pregabalin reduces pain and improves sleep and mood disturbances in patients with post-herpetic neuralgia: results of a randomised, placebo-controlled clinical trial. Pain 2004; 109:26–35.
6. Backonja M, Beydoun A, Edwards KR, et al. Gabapentin for the symptomatic treatment of painful neuropathy in patients with diabetes mellitus: a randomized controlled trial. JAMA 1998; 280:1831–1836.
7. Dallocchio C, Buffa C, Mazzarello P, Chiroli S. Gabapentin vs. amitriptyline in painful diabetic neuropathy: an open-label pilot study. J Pain Symptom Manage 2000; 20:280–285.

8. Rowbotham M, Harden N, Stacey B, et al. Gabapentin for the treatment of postherpetic neuralgia: randomized controlled trial. JAMA 1998; 280:1837–1842.

9. Rice AS, Maton S. Gabapentin in postherpetic neuralgia: a randomised, double blind, placebo controlled study. Pain 2001; 94:215–224.

10. Berry JD, Petersen KL. A single dose of gabapentin reduces acute pain and allodynia in patients with herpes zoster. Neurology 2005; 9:444–447.

11. Levendoglu F, Ogün CO, Ozerbil O, et al. Gabapentin is a first line drug for the treatment of neuropathic pain in spinal cord injury. Spine 2004; 29:743–751.

12. Solak O, Metin M, Esme H, et al. Effectiveness of gabapentin in the treatment of chronic post-thoracotomy pain. Eur J Cardiothorac Surg 2007; 32:9–12.

13. Yaksi A, Ozgönenel L, Ozgönenel B. The efficiency of gabapentin therapy in patients with lumbar spinal stenosis. Spine 2007; 32:939–942.

14. Mellick GA, Mellick LB. Gabapentin in the management of reflex sympathetic dystrophy. J Pain Symptom Manage 1995; 10:265–266.

15. La Spina I, Porazzi D, Maggiolo F, et al. Gabapentin in painful HIV-related neuropathy: a report of 19 patients, preliminary observations. Eur J Neurol 2001; 8:71–75.

16. Solaro C, Lunardi GL, Capello E, et al. An open-label trial of gabapentin treatment of paroxysmal symptoms in multiple sclerosis patients. Neurology 1998; 51:609–611.

17. Morello CM, Leckband SG, Stoner CP, et al. Randomized double-blind study comparing the efficacy of gabapentin with amitriptyline on diabetic peripheral neuropathy pain. Arch Int Med 1999; 159:1931–1937.

18. Chandra K, Shafiq N, Pandhi P, et al. Gabapentin versus nortriptyline in post-herpetic neuralgia patients: a randomized, double-blind clinical trial—the GONIP trial. Int J Clin Pharmacol Ther 2006; 44:358–363.

19. Arnold LM, Goldenberg DL, Stanford SB, et al. Gabapentin in the treatment of fibromyalgia: a randomized, double-blind, placebo-controlled, multicenter trial. Arthritis Rheum 2007; 56:1336–1344.

20. Chen C, Han CH, Sweeney M, Cowles VE. Pharmacokinetics, efficacy, and tolerability of a once-daily gastroretentive dosage form of gabapentin for the treatment of postherpetic neuralgia. J Pharm Sci 2013; 102:1155–1164.

21. Jensen MP, Irving G, Rauck R, et al. Long-term safety of gastroretentive gabapentin in postherpetic neuralgia patients. Clin J Pain 2013; 29:770–774.

22. Zhang L, Rainka M, Freeman R, et al. A randomized, double-blind, placebo-controlled trial to assess the efficacy and safety of gabapentin enacarbil in subjects with neuropathic pain associated with postherpetic neuralgia (PXN110748). J Pain 2013; 14:590–603.

23. Harden RN, Kaye AD, Kintanar T, Argoff CE. Evidence-based guidance for the management of postherpetic neuralgia in primary care. Postgrad Med 2013; 125:191–202.

24. Freeman R, Durso-Decruz E, Emir B. Efficacy, safety and tolerability of pregabalin treatment of painful diabetic peripheral neuropathy: findings from 7 randomized, controlled trials across a range of doses. Diabetes Care 2008; 31:1448–1454.

25. Rosenstock J, Tuchman M, LaMoreaux L, Sharma U. Pregabalin for the treatment of painful diabetic peripheral neuropathy: a double-blind, placebo-controlled trial. Pain 2004; 110:628–638.

26. Siddall PJ, Cousins MJ, Otte A, et al. Pregabalin in central neuropathic pain associated with spinal cord injury: a placebo-controlled trial. Neurology 2006; 67:1792–1800.

27. Stacey BR, Dworkin RH, Murphy K, et al. Pregabalin in the treatment of refractory neuropathic pain: results of a 15-month open-label trial. Pain Med 2008; 9:1202–1208.

28. Ney JP, Devine EB, Watanabe JH, Sullivan SD. Comparative efficacy of oral pharmaceuticals for the treatment of chronic peripheral neuropathic pain: meta-analysis and indirect treatment comparisons. Pain Med 2013; 14:706–719.

29. Talukdar R, Reddy DN. Pain in chronic pancreatitis: managing beyond the pancreatic duct. World J Gastroenterol 2013; 19:6319–6328.

30. Nasser K, Kivitz AJ, Maricic MJ, et al. Twice daily versus once nightly dosing of pregabalin for fibromyalgia: a double-blind randomized clinical trial of efficacy and safety. Arthritis Care Res (Hoboken) 2014; 66:293–300.

31. Atalay H, Solak Y, Biyik Z, et al. Cross-over, open-label trial of the effects of gabapentin versus pregabalin on painful peripheral neuropathy and health-related quality of life in haemodialysis patients. Clin Drug Investig 2013; 33:401–408.

32. Carmichael NM, Katz J, Clarke H, et al. An intensive perioperative regimen of pregabalin and celecoxib reduces pain and improves physical function scores six weeks after total hip arthroplasty: a prospective randomized controlled trial. Pain Res Manage 2013; 18:127–132.

33. Chaparro LE, Smith LA, Moore RA, et al. Pharmacotherapy for the prevention of chronic pain after surgery in adults. Cochrane Database Syst Rev 2013 Jul 24; Available at: http://onlinelibrary.wiley.com/doi/10.1002/14651858.CD008307.pub2/abstract. Accessed 19 November, 2014.

34. Fuzier R, Serres I, Guitton E, et al. Adverse drug reactions to gabapentin and pregabalin: a review of the French pharmacovigilance database. Drug Saf 2013; 36:55–62.

35. Wiffen PJ, Derry S, Moore R, et al. Antiepileptic drugs to treat neuropathic pain or fibromyalgia-an overview of Cochrane reviews. Cochrane Database Syst Rev 2013 Nov 11; Available at: http://onlinelibrary.wiley.com/doi/10.1002/14651858.CD010567.pub2/abstract. Accessed 19 November, 2014.

36. Dworkin RH, O'Connor AB, Backonja M, et al. Pharmacologic management of neuropathic pain: evidence-based recommendations. Pain 2007; 132:237–251.

37. Killian JM, Fromm GH. Carbamazepine in the treatment of neuralgia. Use and side effects. Arch Neurol 1968; 19:129–136.

38. Rull JA, Quibrera R, Gonzalez-Millan H, Lozano Castaneda O. Symptomatic treatment of peripheral diabetic neuropathy with carbamazepine (Tegretol): double-blind cross-over trial. Diabetologia 1969; 5:215–218.

39. Dogra S, Beydoun S, Mazzola J, et al. Oxcarbazepine in painful diabetic neuropathy: a randomized, placebo-controlled study. Eur J Pain 2005; 9:543–554.

40. Criscuolo S, Auletta C, Lippi S, et al. Oxcarbazepine monotherapy in postherpetic neuralgia unresponsive to carbamazepine and gabapentin. Acta Neurol Scand 2005; 111:229–232.

41. Zhou M, Chen N, He L, et al. Oxcarbazepine for neuropathic pain. Cochrane Database Syst Rev 2013; Available at: http://onlinelibrary.wiley.com/store/10.1002/14651858.CD007963.pub2/asset/CD007963.pdf?v=1&t=

i2qwqztu&s=4ea02141550c8c53d249f0c406185fa5f97598e2. Accessed 19 November, 2014.

42. Wiffen PJ, Derry S, Moore RA. Lamotrigine for chronic neuropathic pain and fibromyalgia in adults. Cochrane Database Syst Rev 2013; Available at: http://onlinelibrary.wiley.com/doi/10.1002/14651858.CD006044.pub4/pdf. Accessed 19 November, 2014.

43. Thienel U, Neto W, Schwabe SK, et al. Topiramate in painful diabetic polyneuropathy: findings from three double-blind placebo-controlled trials. Acta Neurol Scand 2004; 110:221–231.

44. Muehlbacher M, Nickel MK, Kettler C, et al. Topiramate in treatment of patients with chronic low back pain: a randomized, double-blind, placebo-controlled study. Clin J Pain 2006; 22:526–531.

45. Khoromi S, Patsalides A, Parada S, et al. Topiramate in chronic lumbar radicular pain. J Pain 2005; 6:829–836.

46. Erdogan C, Yücel M, Akgün H, et al. Effects of topiramate on peripheral nerve excitability. J Clin Neurophysiol 2012; 29:268–270.

47. Wiffen PJ, Derry S, Lunn MP, Moore SA. Topiramate for neuropathic pain and fibromyalgia in adults. Available at: http://onlinelibrary.wiley.com/store/10.1002/14651858.CD008314.pub3/asset/CD008314.pdf?v=1&t=i2qx837z&s=551fcba05d2d31f12980e9a8f65348fbbb8f86bd. Accessed 19 November, 2014.

48. Jungehulsing GJ, Israel H, Safar N, et al. Levetiracetam in patients with central neuropatic post-stroke pain—a randomized, double-blind, placebo-controlled trial. Eur J Neurol 2013; 20:331–337.

49. Falah M, Madsen C, Holbech JV, Sindrup SH. A randomized, placebo-controlled trial of levetiracetam in central pain in multiple sclerosis. Eur J Pain 2012; 16:860–869.

50. Holbech JV, Otto M, Bach FW, et al. The anticonvulsant levetiracetam for the treatment of pain in polyneuropathy: a randomized, placebo-controlled, cross-over trial. Eur J Pain 2011; 15:608–614.

51. Hearn L, Derry S, Moore SA. Lacosamide for neuropathic pain and fibromyalgia in adults. Cochrane Database Syst Rev 2012 Feb 15.

52. Atli A, Dogra S. Zonisamide in the treatment of painful diabetic neuropathy: a randomized, doubled-blind, placebo-controlled pilot study. Pain Med 2005; 6:225–234.

Chapter 5

Cannabinoids

Julie Desroches and Pierre Beaulieu

In several countries, such as Canada, and in some states in the United States of America, the use of marihuana (marijuana, cannabis) is authorized for medical purposes. However, cannabis remains illegal throughout the United States and is not approved for prescription as medicine; however, 18 states—Alaska, Arizona, California, Colorado, Connecticut, Delaware, Hawaii, Maine, Massachusetts, Michigan, Montana, Nevada, New Jersey, New Mexico, Oregon, Rhode Island, Vermont, and Washington, as well as the District of Columbia—approve and regulate its medical use*. The Federal government continues to enforce its prohibition in these states. In Canada, the seedlings are produced and delivered by Health Canada with a special medical authorization. Marijuana inhalation exposes the user to many chemical compounds including approximately 70 different phytocannabinoids (Δ9-tetrahydrocannabinol [Δ9-THC], cannabinol, cannabidiol (CBD), cannabigerol, cannabichromene, tetrahydrocannabivarin, etc). In addition to the whole plant, there are synthetic compounds available for prescription such as Δ9-THC or synthetic derivatives (Table 5.1). The distributed dried marijuana has a content of 12.5 ± 2% Δ9-THC. Cannabinoid-based medicines have been evaluated in several clinical trials for their potential role in the treatment of different pain conditions. After a rapid presentation of the cannabinoid system, the role of cannabinoids in various pain conditions is presented.

The cannabinoid system

Since the identification of the principal psychoactive component of cannabis, many data suggest that the cannabinoid system is implicated in pain modulation via the activation of two cloned G-protein coupled receptors ($G_{i/o}$, inhibiting type), cannabinoid receptor (CB)$_1$ and CB$_2$ receptors [1]. The CB receptors are mainly localized in the central nervous system, and they are also found along the pain pathways (primary afferent fibers and spinal cord). By contrast, CB$_2$ receptor expression seems to be found predominantly, but not exclusively, in peripheral tissues with immune functions, although they were also detected in the brain, dorsal root ganglia, lumbar spinal cord, on sensory neurons, on microglia, and in peripheral tissues. Endogenous compounds such as anandamide and 2-arachidonoyl glycerol form the basis of the endocannabinoid system (Figure 5.1). Modulation of the endocannabinoid

* http://medicalmarijuana.procon.org/view.resource.php?resourceID=000881 (accessed 25 March 2013)

Table 5.1 Cannabis-Based Medicines Available in Clinical Practice

Cannabinoids	Aspect	Indications	Posology	Commercial Name	Remarks
Marijuana	Plant	Mostly in chronic pain	Individual	—	In Canada, requires a special medical authorization from Health Canada
Dronabinol	2.5, 5, and 10 mg capsules	Severe nausea and vomiting associated with cancer chemotherapy; AIDS-related anorexia associated with weight loss	2.5 to 5 mg every 12 h max. 20 mg/day	Marinol	Also used in chronic pain management
Nabilone	0.25, 0.5, and 1 mg capsules	Severe nausea and vomiting associated with cancer chemotherapy	1 to 2 mg every 12 h max. 6 mg/day	Cesamet	Also used in chronic pain management
Nabiximols (THC/cannabidiol)	Oromucosal spray containing 2.7 mg THC and 2.5 mg cannabidiol per 100 µL	Adjunctive treatment for the symptomatic relief of neuropathic pain associated with multiple sclerosis and advanced cancer pain	Start with 1 spray every 4 h or less. Average dose: 5 sprays/day	Sativex	Causes irritations in the mouth in 20–25% patients in clinical trials

Abbreviations: AIDS, acquired immune deficiency syndrome; max., maximum; THC, Δ^9-tetrahydrocannabinol.

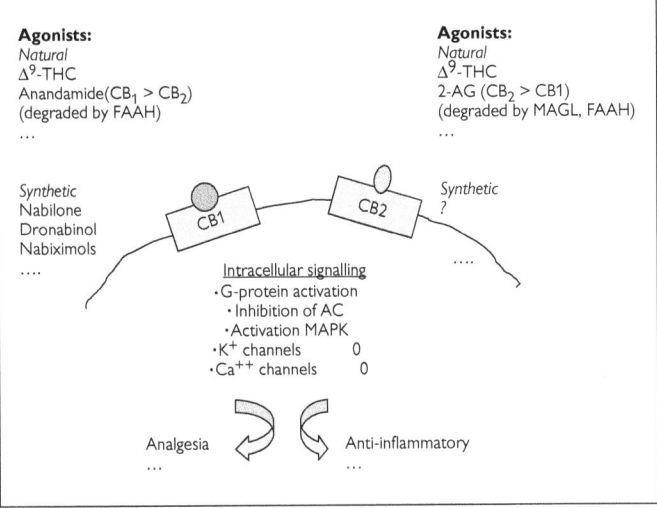

Figure 5.1 Schematic figure illustrating cannabinoid receptor (CB)$_1$ and CB$_2$ receptors and their agonists, and the endocannabinoid (endoCB)-mediated synaptic signaling at glutamatergic synapses. Endocannabinoid signaling is a key regulator of neuronal excitability and both excitatory and inhibitory synaptic transmission throughout the central nervous system. It is regulated by synthesis, release, reuptake, and degradation of endoCBs. (1) Synthesis: endoCB signaling machinery operates on demand in a synapse-specific manner, and endoCBs can be released immediately from postsynaptic neurons. Enzymatic processes can be activated either by membrane depolarization, increases in intracellular calcium levels, or receptor stimulation, leading to the cleavage of membrane phospholipid precursors and subsequent synthesis of endoCBs. (2) Release: endoCBs can act through a retrograde signaling mechanism: released from depolarized postsynaptic neurons into the extracellular space, they can travel to presynaptic terminals, where they can activate cannabinoid receptors and downstream signalization cascade leading to analgesic and anti-inflammatory effects. In this figure illustrating a glutamatergic synapse, endoCBs can inhibit the release of the excitatory neurotransmitter glutamate, thus temporarily inhibiting glutamatergic excitatory post-synaptic currents. (3) Reuptake of endoCBs, and most notably anandamide (AEA), in the synaptic space have been recently shown to be facilitated by a specific transporter. The existence of similar mechanisms for 2-arachidonoylglycerol (2-AG) transport remains controversial. (4) Degradation: the synthesis and metabolism of AEA and 2-AG are controlled by distinct enzymatic pathways. Anandamide is hydrolyzed by the enzyme fatty acid amide hydrolase (FAAH) in postsynaptic neurons, producing ethanolamine and arachidonic acid, whereas 2-AG is degraded, predominantly but not exclusively, by a distinct enzyme monoacylglycerol lipase (MGL) in presynaptic neurons, generating glycerol and arachidonic acid. Δ^9-THC, Δ^9-tetrahydrocannabinol; mGluR$_5$, type 1 metabotropic glutamate receptors.

system has been recently reviewed [2], indicating a significant role for the endocannabinoid system in various pain conditions.

Acute pain

Cannabinoids have shown great efficacy in numerous animal models of acute and inflammatory pain. However, they are least effective in alleviating acute pain in human volunteers and in the postoperative setting. Indeed, in healthy volunteers who were administered cannabinoids, only a few studies have demonstrated an analgesic effect [3, 4]. Despite this negative outcome, it is important to note that in this setting of volunteer studies using noxious heat and inflammatory stimuli, even potent and effective drugs such as opioids often cannot achieve significant pain management [5]. Moreover, there are only four published reports on the use of cannabinoids in postoperative pain, concluding that cannabinoids administration is not appropriate to treat postoperative pain and have either moderate effects [6, 7], no effects different from placebo [8], or even antianalgesic effects at high doses [9]. However, a large multicenter study recruiting patients undergoing operations with a reproducible painful condition and using appropriate dosage is needed before a conclusion can be drawn on the effect of cannabinoids in acute postoperative pain management.

Chronic pain

In general, cannabinoids are moderately effective for the treatment of chronic pain conditions [10]. Several recent studies using a substantial number of patients have shown that cannabinoids were effective in relieving pain in patients suffering from several types of chronic pain, such as neuropathic pain (including human immunodeficiency virus [HIV] neuropathic pain), spinal cord injury (SCI), pain associated with multiple sclerosis (MS), musculoskeletal disorders, fibromyalgia, or other chronic pain conditions (for a review, see [11, 12]).

Neuropathic pain

Several randomized, placebo-controlled, double-blind, crossover and parallel studies have evaluated cannabinoids for the relief of central or peripheral neuropathic pain (see also Chapter 9.1). Overall, cannabinoids had modest but significant analgesic effects often associated with adverse effects in the treatment of neuropathic pain states. Patients suffering from neuropathic pain of different etiologies reported benefits after treatment with Δ^9-THC/CBD concomitantly with other analgesic drugs [13–16]. However, negative outcomes were reported by two trials among neuropathic pain patients using dronabinol and nabilone [17, 18].

Numerous clinical trials have examined the efficacy of smoked cannabis for neuropathic pain. For example, one randomized, placebo-controlled, crossover trial performed in 38 patients reported significant decreases in central and peripheral neuropathic pain when using smoked cannabis [19]. More recently, a randomized, placebo-controlled study evaluated smoked cannabis among 21 patients suffering from posttraumatic or postsurgical neuropathic pain refractory to conventional therapies [20]. Patients reported that after a single inhalation of 25 mg of 9.4% Δ9-THC herbal cannabis three times daily for five days, there was a modest but statistically significant reduction in average daily pain intensity, with significant improvements in sleep quality and anxiety [20].

Smoked cannabis also exerts antinociceptive effects compared with placebo in HIV-associated neuropathic pain patients, according to two studies that reported a greater than 30% reduction in pain [21] and a 30% decrease in HIV-associated sensory neuropathic pain in patients smoking cannabis [22]. However, medical utilization of smoked marijuana may be limited by its method of administration (smoking) and modest acute cognitive effects, predominantly at higher doses. The issue of whether smoked cannabis should be used in clinical practice is controversial, with supporters arguing that it is premature to claim that there is no future for smoked medical marijuana [23], and some opponents are not convinced of its future in a clinical setting [24]. The recent development of vaporizers to inhale cannabis may decrease its toxicity compared with smoked cannabis, although it remains to be demonstrated in adequately designed clinical studies.

In conclusion, there is some clinical evidence supporting cannabinoids as a treatment of symptoms associated with neuropathic pain and as an important alternative for patients who are not responding to other conventional analgesics.

Spinal cord injury

Although still limited, available clinical data support the findings of preclinical animal studies [25–27] suggesting that cannabinoids could alleviate symptoms associated with neuropathic SCI such as pain, spasticity, muscle spasms, urinary incontinence, and difficulty sleeping. Two double-blinded, placebo-controlled, crossover studies performed in patients suffering from SCI suggested modest improvements in pain, spasticity, muscle spasms, and sleep quality with oral Δ9-THC and/or Δ9-THC/CBD [13, 28]. A randomized, double-blind, placebo-controlled parallel study using Δ9-THC showed a statistically significant improvement in spasticity scores in patients with SCI [29]. Moreover, a recent double-blind, placebo-controlled, crossover study performed in 12 patients with SCI reported improved Asworth (spasticity) scores compared with placebo after a treatment with nabilone (0.5 mg b.i.d.) for 4 weeks [30]. Although no definitive clinical conclusions can be made, these studies suggest a potential benefit of cannabinoids in patients suffering from SCI.

Multiple sclerosis

Preclinical studies and many clinical studies support cannabinoids use to alleviate symptoms associated with MS (reviewed in Ref. [31]). Accordingly, mostly all clinical trials devoted to the use of cannabinoids in pain and spasticity treatment associated with MS were positive. For example, the Cannabis in Multiple Sclerosis (CAMS) study, a large multicentre, randomized, placebo-controlled trial, evaluated oral cannabis extracts Δ^9-THC/CBD, oral Δ^9-THC, or a placebo for 15 weeks in 630 patients suffering from MS. Subjective pain scores and spasticity were significantly better in the cannabinoids group, but there was no difference in the overall spasticity scores using the Ashworth scale [32]. Other randomized clinical studies using cannabis extract Δ9-THC/CBD [33, 34] and standardized cannabis extract capsules [35] reported similar results, with subjective improvements of spasticity not confirmed by objective measures.

Nevertheless, a CAMS follow-up study showed a small long-term treatment effect of oral Δ9-THC on muscle spasticity measures by the Asworth scale [36], and a long-term, open-label, follow-up study using Δ9-THC/CBD concluded that positive effects were maintained in patients who had initially perceived benefits [37]. Two other studies (a randomized, double-blind, placebo-controlled, parallel-group trial and its extension) performed in patients suffering from central neuropathic pain associated with MS revealed that the oromucosal cannabis extract Δ^9-THC/CBD was effective in reducing pain and sleep disturbances with a good adverse effects profile [38, 39]. Moreover, a randomized, double-blind, placebo-controlled, crossover trial concluded that an administration of 10 mg of dronabinol had a modest but clinically relevant analgesic effect on central pain in patients with MS, with a pain reduction similar to traditional analgesics [40]. Overall, although results seem to be clinically significant mostly on subjective measures, cannabinoids may be effective to relieve MS associated pain (for a review, see Ref. [41]).

Musculoskeletal pain

Cannabinoids may have a role in the alleviation of symptoms associated with rheumatoid arthritis, as suggested by the identification of a functional endocannabinoid system in the knee synovia of patients suffering from end-stage osteoarthritis and rheumatoid arthritis [42] (see also Chapter 9.3). A randomized, double-blinded, placebo-controlled, multicentre parallel group study performed in 58 patients suffering from rheumatoid arthritis indicated that a Δ^9-THC/CBD extract administered for five weeks was a modest but statistically significant analgesic for pain on movement and at rest, and it also exerted benefits on quality of sleep with outcomes favoring cannabis over placebo [43]. Another study involving patients suffering from refractory musculoskeletal pain [44] showed that nabilone had significant analgesic effects compared with placebo. However, according to a recent review, there is currently weak evidence that oromucosal cannabis is superior to placebo in reducing pain in patients suffering from rheumatoid arthritis [45].

Fibromyalgia

In some diseases, cannabinoids might be effective in only a subpopulation of patients suffering from that disease. For example, an open-label pilot study performed in patients suffering from fibromyalgia examined the effect of dronabinol on experimentally induced pain, axon reflex flare, and pain relief and reported that only some patients experienced significant pain relief, with a high dose [46]. However, intolerable adverse effects caused a high rate of patient dropout. A randomized, double-blind, placebo-controlled trial was performed in 40 patients suffering from fibromyalgia [47] with nabilone 1 mg b.i.d. for four consecutive weeks. Patients subjectively reported significant improvements in pain relief and anxiety, as well as in Fibromyalgia Impact Questionnaire scores. However, nabilone treatment did not attenuate the number of tender points nor the tender point pain threshold, and it did not retain any lasting benefit after its discontinuation. A multicenter retrospective study also suggested cannabinoids effectiveness in fibromyalgia, but the study suffered from considerable limitations hampering its credibility [48]. Patients on an average daily dose of 7.5 mg of Δ9-THC reported a significant decrease in pain scores, depression symptoms, and intake of concomitant medications such as opioids after an average treatment period of seven months. A recent cross-sectional study of patients with fibromyalgia using self-administered cannabis reported significant benefits in pain, stiffness, relaxation, somnolence, and well being associated with tolerable adverse effects [49]. Unfortunately, the study suffered from many limitations, making its interpretation problematic. Overall, there is insufficient clinical data to endorse cannabis or cannabinoids for the treatment of fibromyalgia.

Cancer pain

Four studies performed more than 34 years ago have valued cannabinoids potential for cancer-related pain treatment. The first two studies are randomized, double-blind, placebo-controlled trials evaluating the analgesic effectiveness of oral Δ^9-THC (dronabinol) in patients suffering from moderate to severe refractory cancer pain. The first study was performed in 10 cancer patients treated with an escalating dose of 5, 10, 15, and 20 mg Δ^9-THC [50]. Patients reported significant pain relief with the two higher doses but unfortunately also experienced severe adverse effects. The second study was performed in 36 cancer patients comparing 10 and 20 mg Δ^9-THC with 60 and 120 mg of codeine [51]. Patients reported mild analgesic effects, but Δ9-THC highest dose induced somnolence, dizziness, ataxia, and blurred vision. However, authors concluded that a 10 mg Δ9-THC regimen, despite its sedative effect, seemed to have analgesic potential in these patients. Adverse effects apparently interfered with cannabinoids benefits in this context. Indeed, another study tested a nitrogen analog of Δ9-THC in cancer patients and reported that although pain relief was superior to placebo and approximately equivalent to 50 mg of codeine phosphate, the synthetic analog was not considered clinically useful because of the adverse effects profile [52]. In contrast, a study comparing a Δ^9-THC nitrogen analog with codeine and placebo in patients suffering from chronic pain due to malignancies demonstrated that benzopyranoperidine (a synthetic analog of Δ^9-THC) did not produce analgesic effects and even seemed to increase pain perception [53].

A recent randomized, double-blinded, placebo-controlled, parallel-group study evaluated a cannabis extract (Δ^9-THC/CBD), a Δ^9-THC extract, and placebo in 177 patients suffering from intractable cancer-associated pain not fully relieved by strong opioids [54]. Approximately 43% of patients subjectively reported a 30% or greater improvement in pain score, which was twice the number of patients who achieved this response in the Δ^9-THC and placebo groups. Both cannabinoid regimens were well tolerated, and adverse effects were mild to moderate (somnolence, dizziness, and nausea).

Additional clinical trials evaluating the therapeutic efficacy of cannabinoids in cancer pain are needed, especially given cannabinoids additional therapeutic potential regarding antiemetic and antitumour properties (for a review, see Ref. [55]).

Adverse effects of cannabinoids

The most common adverse effects of cannabinoids are related to their actions on the central nervous system and include euphoria, dysphoria, anxiety, drowsiness, amnesia, psychomotor retardation, and cognitive impairment (Table 5.2). Although possible, psychosis is relatively rare. These adverse effects are reversible upon discontinuation of the cannabinoids. Adverse effects on cardiovascular, reproductive, pulmonary, and immune systems have also been reported. No death related to overdose has been reported. Development of dependency to cannabinoids has been reported in 10% of patients treated with cannabinoids [56]. These adverse effects are the main drawbacks to patient compliance with therapy [10], and significant obstacles remain before achieving clinically relevant outcomes with minimal adverse effects. More data is therefore required on the long-term adverse effects of cannabinoid therapy, including drug interactions, tolerance, cognitive impairment, and risks of addiction. High-quality trials with long-term exposure are required to further characterize safety issues related to the use of medical cannabinoids [57].

Opioids-cannabinoids interactions

Because cannabinoids and opioids are distinct drug classes with different effects on pain modulation and pain-relieving mechanisms, there has been considerable clinical interest in investigating combinations of different opioids and cannabinoids to enhance the potency of both compounds.

Some clinical reports support the use of combined administration of cannabinoids and opioids for peripheral inflammatory pain, acute pain, and chronic pain in human volunteers. In addition, a study has examined the effect of adding a cannabinoid to the regimen of patients experiencing chronic pain despite taking stable doses of opioids and has concluded that dronabinol may be a useful adjuvant analgesic for these patients (for a review, see Ref. [58]). Moreover, a recent clinical trial was performed in 21 patients suffering from chronic pain using inhaled vaporized cannabis concomitantly with sustained-release morphine or oxycodone. The authors concluded that cannabis augments analgesia in patients already on a stable opioid regimen without significantly altering plasma opioid levels or metabolism [59].

Overall, opioid and cannabinoid interactions may lead to additive or even synergistic antinociceptive effects, emphasizing their clinical relevance in humans in order to reduce requirements for opioids.

Conclusions on cannabinoids as adjuvant analgesics

Although preclinical evidence highlights the importance of cannabinoid receptors in controlling nociceptive transmission, data obtained from clinical trials are less conclusive regarding the analgesic efficacy of smoked marijuana and synthetic cannabinoids [60, 61]. In acute pain trials, negative or equivocal

Table 5.2 Moderate to Severe Cannabis Adverse Effects On Different Systems

Central Nervous System
- Euphoria, dysphoria
- Anxiety/nervousness
- Amnesia, confusion, depersonalization
- Drowsiness, dizziness, somnolence
- Transient impairment of sensory and perceptual functions
- Psychomotor retardation
- Cognitive impairments
- Depression, amotivational syndrome, psychosis, schizophrenia

Respiratory Tract
- Decreased pulmonary function
- Chronic obstructive airway diseases
- Pulmonary infections

Immune System
- Immunomodulatory/immunosuppressive effects

Reproductive and Endocrine System
- Reduced neonatal birth weight and length
- Slightly increased risk of sudden infant death
- Decline in sperm count, concentration and motility
- Increase in abnormal sperm morphology

Cardiovascular System
- Dose-related tachycardia
- Fluctuations in blood pressure
- Coronary insufficiency
- Myocardial infarction
- Peripheral vasodilation, postural hypotension, and characteristic conjunctival reddening

Liver
- Implication in chronic liver diseases
- Association with moderate to severe fibrosis

Carcinogenesis and Mutagenesis
- Mutagenic effects
- Precancerous pulmonary pathology

Tolerance, Dependence and Abuse
- Dependence in 1 out of 10 people
- Behaviors of preoccupation, compulsion, reinforcement, and withdrawal

Overdose/Toxicity
- No documented evidence of death directly attributable to cannabis overdose

results have been reported with the use of cannabis or cannabinoid-based medicines. The best evidence for an analgesic efficacy of cannabinoids is for neuropathic pain associated with MS, but evidence is also accumulating for other types of chronic pain. However, scientific studies supporting the analgesic activity and safety of smoked cannabis are still limited and generally inconclusive. Thus, further large clinical trials evaluating smoked marijuana in clinical practice are mandatory.

Overall, the publication of several important clinical studies emphasizing the potential role for cannabinoids in pain management and ongoing work on the subject make cannabinoids worthy of consideration as an adjuvant analgesic for refractory pain conditions. Clinicians working in pain management should be aware of the options becoming available from the cannabinoid class of medications because international guidelines for the treatment of neuropathic pain have included cannabinoids in their algorithm, not as a first-line treatment but as a third or fourth option [62]. However, it is still crucial to fully inform patients of the adverse-effect profile associated with the use of cannabinoids and to monitor the patients carefully.

References

1. Guindon J, Hohmann AG, Beaulieu P. Pharmacology of the cannabinoid system. In: Beaulieu P, Lussier D, Porreca F, Dickenson AH, eds. *Pharmacology of Pain*: IASP Press, Seattle; 2010: pp. 111–138.

2. Guindon J, Hohmann AG. The endocannabinoid system and pain. CNS Neurol Disord Drug Targets 2009; 8:403–421.

3. Redmond WJ, Goffaux P, Potvin S, et al. Analgesic and antihyperalgesic effects of nabilone on experimental heat pain. Curr Med Res Opin 2008; 24:1017–1024.

4. Rukwied R, Watkinson A, McGlone F, et al. Cannabinoid agonists attenuate capsaicin-induced responses in human skin. Pain 2003; 102:283–288.

5. Naef M, Curatolo M, Petersen-Felix S, et al. The analgesic effect of oral delta-9-tetrahydrocannabinol (THC), morphine, and a THC-morphine combination in healthy subjects under experimental pain conditions. Pain 2003; 105:79–88.

6. Jain AK, Ryan JR, McMahon FG, et al. Evaluation of intramuscular levonantradol and placebo in acute postoperative pain. J Clin Pharmacol 1981; 21(8–9 Suppl):320S–326S.

7. Holdcroft A, Maze M, Dore C, et al. A multicenter dose-escalation study of the analgesic and adverse effects of an oral cannabis extract (Cannador) for postoperative pain management. Anesthesiology 2006; 104:1040–1046.

8. Buggy DJ, Toogood L, Maric S, et al. Lack of analgesic efficacy of oral delta-9-tetrahydrocannabinol in postoperative pain. Pain 2003; 106:169–172.

9. Beaulieu P. Effects of nabilone, a synthetic cannabinoid, on postoperative pain. Can J Anaesth 2006; 53:769–775.

10. Beaulieu P, Ware M. Reassessment of the role of cannabinoids in the management of pain. Curr Opin Anaesthesiol 2007; 20:473–477.

11. Martin-Sanchez E, Furukawa TA, Taylor J, et al. Systematic review and meta-analysis of cannabis treatment for chronic pain. Pain Med 2009; 10:1353–1368.

12. Lynch ME, Campbell F. Cannabinoids for treatment of chronic non-cancer pain; a systematic review of randomized trials. Br J Clin Pharmacol 2011; 72:735–744.

13. Wade DT, Robson P, House H, et al. A preliminary controlled study to determine whether whole-plant cannabis extracts can improve intractable neurogenic symptoms. Clin Rehabil 2003; 17:21–29.

14. Berman JS, Symonds C, Birch R. Efficacy of two cannabis based medicinal extracts for relief of central neuropathic pain from brachial plexus avulsion: results of a randomised controlled trial. Pain 2004; 112:299–306.

15. Notcutt W, Price M, Miller R, et al. Initial experiences with medicinal extracts of cannabis for chronic pain: results from 34 "N of 1" studies. Anaesthesia 2004; 59:440–452.

16. Nurmikko TJ, Serpell MG, Hoggart B, et al. Sativex successfully treats neuropathic pain characterised by allodynia: a randomised, double-blind, placebo-controlled clinical trial. Pain 2007; 133:210–220.

17. Attal N, Brasseur L, Guirimand D, et al. Are oral cannabinoids safe and effective in refractory neuropathic pain? Eur J Pain 2004; 8:173–177.

18. Frank B, Serpell MG, Hughes J, et al. Comparison of analgesic effects and patient tolerability of nabilone and dihydrocodeine for chronic neuropathic pain: randomised, crossover, double blind study. BMJ 2008; 336:199–201.

19. Wilsey B, Marcotte T, Tsodikov A, et al. A randomized, placebo-controlled, crossover trial of cannabis cigarettes in neuropathic pain. J Pain 2008; 9:506–521.

20. Ware MA, Wang T, Shapiro S, et al. Smoked cannabis for chronic neuropathic pain: a randomized controlled trial. CMAJ 2010; 182:E694–E701.

21. Abrams DI, Jay CA, Shade SB, et al. Cannabis in painful HIV-associated sensory neuropathy: a randomized placebo-controlled trial. Neurology 2007; 68:515–521.

22. Ellis RJ, Toperoff W, Vaida F, et al. Smoked medicinal cannabis for neuropathic pain in HIV: a randomized, crossover clinical trial. Neuropsychopharmacology 2009; 34:672–680.

23. Ware MA. Clearing the smoke around medical marijuana. Clin Pharmacol Ther 2011; 90:769–771.

24. Kalant H. Smoked marijuana as medicine: not much future. Clin Pharmacol Ther 2008; 83:517–519.

25. Hama A, Sagen J. Antinociceptive effect of cannabinoid agonist WIN 55,212-2 in rats with a spinal cord injury. Exp Neurol 2007; 204:454–457.

26. Hama A, Sagen J. Sustained antinociceptive effect of cannabinoid receptor agonist WIN 55,212-2 over time in rat model of neuropathic spinal cord injury pain. J Rehabil Res Dev 2009; 46:135–143.

27. Garcia-Ovejero D, Arevalo-Martin A, Petrosino S, et al. The endocannabinoid system is modulated in response to spinal cord injury in rats. Neurobiol Dis 2009; 33:57–71.

28. Maurer M, Henn V, Dittrich A, et al. Delta-9-tetrahydrocannabinol shows antispastic and analgesic effects in a single case double-blind trial. Eur Arch Psychiatry Clin Neurosci 1990; 240:1–4.

29. Hagenbach U, Luz S, Ghafoor N, et al. The treatment of spasticity with Delta9-tetrahydrocannabinol in persons with spinal cord injury. Spinal Cord 2007; 45:551–562.

30. Pooyania S, Ethans K, Szturm T, et al. A randomized, double-blinded, crossover pilot study assessing the effect of nabilone on spasticity in persons with spinal cord injury. Arch Phys Med Rehabil 2010; 91:703–707.

31. Pertwee RG. Cannabinoids and multiple sclerosis. Mol Neurobiol 2007; 36:45–59.

32. Zajicek J, Fox P, Sanders H, et al. Cannabinoids for treatment of spasticity and other symptoms related to multiple sclerosis (CAMS study): multicentre randomised placebo-controlled trial. Lancet 2003; 362:1517–1526.

33. Wade DT, Makela P, Robson P, et al. Do cannabis-based medicinal extracts have general or specific effects on symptoms in multiple sclerosis? A double-blind, randomized, placebo-controlled study on 160 patients. Mult Scler 2004; 10:434–441.

34. Collin C, Davies P, Mutiboko IK, et al. Randomized controlled trial of cannabis-based medicine in spasticity caused by multiple sclerosis. Eur J Neurol 2007; 14:290–296.

35. Vaney C, Heinzel-Gutenbrunner M, Jobin P, et al. Efficacy, safety and tolerability of an orally administered cannabis extract in the treatment of spasticity in patients with multiple sclerosis: a randomized, double-blind, placebo-controlled, crossover study. Mult Scler 2004; 10:417–424.

36. Zajicek JP, Sanders HP, Wright DE, et al. Cannabinoids in multiple sclerosis (CAMS) study: safety and efficacy data for 12 months follow up. J Neurol Neurosurg Psychiatry 2005; 76:1664–1669.

37. Wade DT, Makela PM, House H, et al. Long-term use of a cannabis-based medicine in the treatment of spasticity and other symptoms in multiple sclerosis. Mult Scler 2006; 12:639–645.

38. Rog DJ, Nurmikko TJ, Friede T, et al. Randomized, controlled trial of cannabis-based medicine in central pain in multiple sclerosis. Neurology 2005; 65:812–819.

39. Rog DJ, Nurmikko TJ, Young CA. Oromucosal delta9-tetrahydrocannabinol/cannabidiol for neuropathic pain associated with multiple sclerosis: an uncontrolled, open-label, 2-year extension trial. Clin Ther 2007; 29:2068–2079.

40. Svendsen KB, Jensen TS, Bach FW. Does the cannabinoid dronabinol reduce central pain in multiple sclerosis? Randomised double blind placebo controlled crossover trial. BMJ 2004; 329:253.

41. Zajicek JP, Apostu VI. Role of cannabinoids in multiple sclerosis. CNS Drugs 2011; 25:187–201.

42. Richardson D, Pearson RG, Kurian N, et al. Characterisation of the cannabinoid receptor system in synovial tissue and fluid in patients with osteoarthritis and rheumatoid arthritis. Arthritis Res Ther 2008; 10:R43.

43. Blake DR, Robson P, Ho M, et al. Preliminary assessment of the efficacy, tolerability and safety of a cannabis-based medicine (Sativex) in the treatment of pain caused by rheumatoid arthritis. Rheumatology (Oxford) 2006; 45:50–52.

44. Pinsger M, Schimetta W, Volc D, et al. [Benefits of an add-on treatment with the synthetic cannabinomimetic nabilone on patients with chronic pain—a randomized controlled trial]. Wien Klin Wochenschr 2006; 118:327–335.

45. Richards BL, Whittle SL, Buchbinder R. Neuromodulators for pain management in rheumatoid arthritis. Cochrane Database Syst Rev 2012; 1:CD008921.

46. Schley M, Legler A, Skopp G, et al. Delta-9-THC based monotherapy in fibromyalgia patients on experimentally induced pain, axon reflex flare, and pain relief. Curr Med Res Opin 2006; 22:1269–1276.

47. Skrabek RQ, Galimova L, Ethans K, et al. Nabilone for the treatment of pain in fibromyalgia. J Pain 2008; 9:164–173.

48. Weber J, Schley M, Casutt M, et al. Tetrahydrocannabinol (Delta 9-THC) treatment in chronic central neuropathic pain and fibromyalgia patients: results of a multicenter survey. Anesthesiol Res Pract 2009; 2009.

49. Fiz J, Duran M, Capella D, et al. Cannabis use in patients with fibromyalgia: effect on symptoms relief and health-related quality of life. PLoS One 2011; 6:e18440.

50. Noyes R Jr, Brunk SF, Baram DA, et al. Analgesic effect of delta-9-tetrahydrocannabinol. J Clin Pharmacol 1975; 15:139–143.

51. Noyes R Jr, Brunk SF, Avery DA, et al. The analgesic properties of delta-9-tetrahydrocannabinol and codeine. Clin Pharmacol Ther 1975; 18:84–89.

52. Staquet M, Gantt C, Machin D. Effect of a nitrogen analog of tetrahydrocannabinol on cancer pain. Clin Pharmacol Ther 1978; 23:397–401.

53. Jochimsen PR, Lawton RL, VerSteeg K, et al. Effect of benzopyranoperidine, a delta-9-THC congener, on pain. Clin Pharmacol Ther 1978; 24:223–227.

54. Johnson JR, Burnell-Nugent M, Lossignol D, et al. Multicenter, double-blind, randomized, placebo-controlled, parallel-group study of the efficacy, safety, and tolerability of THC:CBD extract and THC extract in patients with intractable cancer-related pain. J Pain Symptom Manage 2010; 39:167–179.

55. Guindon J, Hohmann AG. The endocannabinoid system and cancer: therapeutic implication. Br J Pharmacol 2011; 163:1447–1463.

56. Lichtman AH, Martin BR. Cannabinoid tolerance and dependence. Handb Exp Pharmacol 2005; 691–717.

57. Wang T, Collet JP, Shapiro S, et al. Adverse effects of medical cannabinoids: a systematic review. CMAJ 2008; 178:1669–1678.

58. Desroches J, Beaulieu P. Opioids and cannabinoids interactions: involvement in pain management. Curr Drug Targets 2010; 11:462–473.

59. Abrams DI, Couey P, Shade SB, et al. Cannabinoid-opioid interaction in chronic pain. Clin Pharmacol Ther 2011; 90:844–851.

60. Hosking RD, Zajicek JP. Therapeutic potential of cannabis in pain medicine. Br J Anaesth 2008; 101:59–68.

61. Leung L. Cannabis and its derivatives: review of medical use. J Am Board Fam Med 2011; 24:452–462.

62. Attal N, Cruccu G, Baron R, et al. EFNS guidelines on the pharmacological treatment of neuropathic pain: 2010 revision. Eur J Neurol 2010; 17:1113–1188.

Chapter 6

Local Anesthetics

Patrick Friederich

Local anesthetics constitute a group of pharmacological agents that are injected into the vicinity of a peripheral nerve or spinal cord. Local and regional anesthesia is widely accepted as being a safe and even beneficial anesthetic technique for pain therapy with a low rate of complications [1]. Clinical use of local anesthetics therefore requires basic knowledge of the anatomy and physiology of peripheral and central pain transmission [2], technical skills in localizing peripheral nerves and in the performance of nerve blocks [3], as well as knowledge of the pharmacologic properties of these drugs [4]. Apart from complications resulting from technical difficulties in performing the nerve block, severe toxic complications result from inadvertent drug effects. With the advent of ultrasound-guided regional anesthetic techniques [5] and lipid rescue therapy [6], the application of local anesthetics has never been as safe. Ultrasound imaging allows the precise injection of local anesthetics directly into the vicinity of peripheral nerves under visual control. This technique helps to reduce the dose of the local anesthetic. Furthermore, physical damage of nerves by the injection needle and inadvertent injection of local anesthetics into blood vessels can also be decreased. Local anesthetics can also be administered systemically or topically for some indications. Treatment protocols have been developed for this clinical use. This chapter offers a pharmacological and neurophysiological approach to the clinical use of a very potent group of extremely beneficial pharmacological agents.

Local anesthetics and the anatomy of pain transmission

Pain sensation results from the activation of specific nociceptive information conducting structures distributed throughout the human body [2]. The nociceptive information is transmitted to the sensory cortex and interpreted as pain by higher brain function. Pharmacological therapy with local anesthetics aims at interrupting the transmission of nociceptive information from the peripheral nervous system to the brain. For this purpose, local anesthetics are applied to the skin or injected into tissue or in the vicinity of peripheral nerves or spinal cord. In a simplistic view, local anesthetics may be considered as blockers of ascending nociceptive information transmitted by afferent neurons from the periphery of the human body to the sensory cortex. Table 6.1 provides an overview of the various routes and techniques of administration of local anesthetics.

Table 6.1 Routes and Techniques of Administration of Local Anesthetics

Topical	• Ophthalmic, otologic: drops
	• Cutaneous: creams (eutectic mixture of local anesthetics), patch, gels, dental paste
	• Mucosa: vaporisation (buccal, pharyngeal, bronchial, gastric, anal, etc)
Incision blocks	• Subcutaneous, subfascial
Intra-articular and bursa blocks	
Neuraxial blocks	• Epidural
	• Rachianesthesia
	• Caudal block
Peripheral nerve and plexus blocks	• Plexus blocks: brachial, lumbosacral
	• Proximal and distal nerve blocks: face, extremities
Parietal blocks	• Intercostal blocks
	• Block of abdominal transverse or transversus abdominis plane block
	• Rectus abdominis block
	• Pectoral block
Other blocks	• Dorsal penile nerve block
	• Paravertebral block

Nociception

The primary afferent neurons involved in pain transmission are called nociceptors. They are activated by noxious stimuli such as mechanical, thermal, or chemical insult threatening tissue integrity. Activation of nociceptors initiates nociception, that is, the transmission of neural information via peripheral nerves and the spinal cord to the brain where this information is interpreted as pain. Infiltration of local anesthetics into human tissue such as the skin aims at preventing pain sensation by blocking activation of nociceptors and blockade of very superficially located peripheral endings of the primary afferent neurons. Infiltration of local anesthetics into the skin or superficial tissue only makes sense if the region of insult is restricted to a very small superficial anatomical region. If nociceptive information is transmitted from larger regions than a small and defined local area, a peripheral nerve block or neuraxial analgesia that covers a larger region of the body needs to be considered [3].

Transmission of nociceptive information by peripheral nerves

Peripheral nerves transmit information from peripheral regions of the human body to the brain. The more distal the nerve is from the brain, the smaller is the anatomic region it transmits information from. The peripheral nerves most frequently blocked by local anesthetics clinically derive from either the brachial plexus or the lumbosacral plexus. Peripheral nerves such as the radial and ulnar nerves or the femoral and the sciatic nerves transmit sensation from the upper and lower extremities, respectively [3]. They are blocked for surgeries on larger parts of a single upper or lower extremity such as surgeries for a fractured arm or leg. If the region of interest is too large for a single or a limited number of nerve blocks, the entire plexus may be approached for blockade by local anesthetics.

Nociceptive information originating in the thoracic region is transmitted by intercostal and subcostal nerves via the dorsal and ventral rami of the spinal nerves to the spinal cord. The muscles and skin of the back of the body are supplied by the dorsal rami of the spinal nerves. Intercostal and subcostal nerves can easily be blocked by local anesthetics. Such blocks may be performed for treatment of postherpetic neuralgia or for alleviating pain resulting from thoracotomy or rib fracture.

Transmission of nociceptive information by the spinal cord

If pain sensation does not result from regions attributable to a single extremity or a limited number of peripheral nerves, nociception may be blocked at the level of the spinal cord [2, 3]. Nerves arriving from different regions of the body converge to nerve columns such as the spinothalamic tract. At the level of the spinal cord, different neurophysiologic information carried by specialized fibers of individual peripheral nerves is distributed into different columns, ascending or descending within the spinal cord to and from the brain. Pain and temperature sensation is transmitted by other columns than those responsible for the transmission of proprioception and motor control.

Systemic application of local anesthetics

Apart from injecting local anesthetics in the vicinity of neural structures, the systemic application of local anesthetics (eg, intravenous lidocaine or oral mexiletine) has been advocated in recent years [7–9]. This application is still of unclear clinical benefit and part of ongoing clinical studies. Promising results with an intravenous infusion of lidocaine have been reported in treating perioperative pain in abdominal surgery and acute pain due to burns, as well as some types of neuropathic pain, including central pain, postherpetic neuralgia, and peripheral diabetic neuropathy. Oral formulations of sodium channel blockers similar to local anesthetics (flecainide, tocainide, mexiletine) have been shown to relieve some types of neuropathic pain. Furthermore, some studies suggest anti-inflammatory action of local anesthetics offering benefits for long-term survival in selected cancer patients [10, 11]; however, these is a lack of sufficient clinical evidence to support widespread recommendations.

Topical application of local anesthetics

A mixture of prilocaine and lignocaine (eutectic mixture of local anesthetics), which penetrates the skin and produces a dense local cutaneous anesthesia, is often used to prevent pain from needle puncture, incision, or debridement of leg ulcers [12]. Limited evidence also suggests efficacy in treating some types of neuropathic pain, including postherpetic neuralgia. High-concentration topical lidocaine and 5% lidocaine gel might also produce local analgesia. A lidocaine 5% patch is often recommended as first-line therapy for treatment of localized neuropathic pain [13].

Local application of local anesthetics does not usually result in systemic absorption, and hence it is not associated with toxicity. However, it should not be applied to open wounds or mucous membranes, and it should only be applied on a limited skin area.

Pharmacology of local anesthetics

Based on pharmacological properties, most local anesthetics can be classified into two groups [4]: amino ester or amino amide local anesthetic. The former group includes drugs such as procaine, chloroprocaine, tetracaine, and cocaine. Frequently used amino amides include lidocaine, mepivacaine, prilocaine, ropivacaine, and bupivacaine. Local anesthetic agents differ in their pharmaceutical structure. From a simplistic view, it is safe to argue that their structural differences strongly influence the onset and duration of action without affecting other pharmacodynamic aspects. Thus, every local anesthetic may be used for local infiltration, peripheral nerve block, or blockade at the level of the spinal cord. Choosing one local anesthetic agent over another is largely determined by the desired onset and duration of therapeutic effect and hence pharmacokinetic considerations. The faster the onset, the shorter the duration of action. The longer the duration, however, the higher the risk of seizure and severe cardiac arrhythmia when inadvertently injected into the systemic circulation.

Most local anesthetics are used as racemic mixtures. Purified isomers of the long-acting amino amides ropivacaine and bupivacaine have been marketed and introduced into clinical practice with the hope to increase the therapeutic safety of long-duration amino amide local anesthetic agents. Whether currently used long-acting local anesthetics at equipotent concentrations significantly differ in their toxicological profile is still a matter of some debate. This debate is largely nourished by the knowledge that both significant clinical advantages as well as toxicological disadvantages result from the same structural properties of the drug molecule.

Anesthetic potency, onset, and duration of action

Hydrophobicity, as determined by the octanol-buffer partition coefficient, seems to be the primary determinant of anesthetic potency, as well as speed of onset and duration of action [4]. The higher the coefficient, the lower the dose needed for the same clinical endpoint, the slower the onset, and the longer the duration of action. This principle is best demonstrated with the homolog series of amino amide local anesthetics mepivacaine, ropivacaine, and bupivacaine. The differences between these drugs result from the different length of their alkyl side chains attached to the aromatic ring (Figure 6.1). The alkyl side chain is a methyl group (mepivacaine), a propyl group (ropivacaine), and a butyl group (bupivacaine), respectively. The hydrophobicity increases with the length of the alkyl side chain as does the potency of the local anesthetic, the speed of onset, as well as the duration of action and, unfortunately, the occurrence of severe neurological and cardiac side effects after inadvertent systemic application. The desired increase

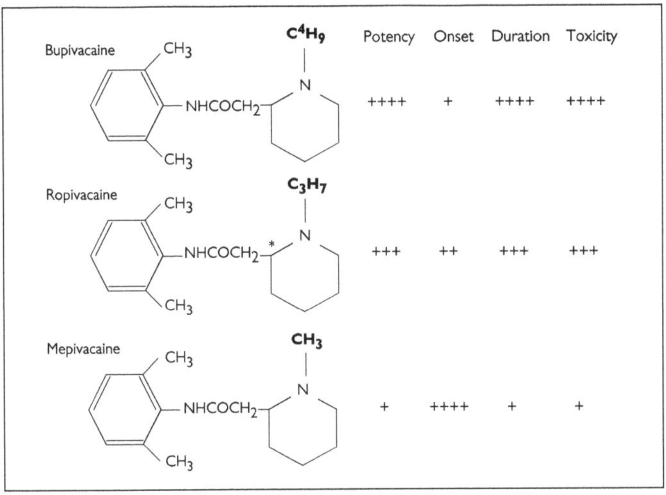

Figure 6.1 Differences in the molecular structure between frequently used amino amide local anesthetics. The alkyl side chain is a methyl group (mepivacaine), a propyl group (ropivacaine), and a butyl group (bupivacaine). Hydrophobicity increases with the length of the alkyl side chain.

in anesthetic potency and duration of action is paid for by an increased risk of severe side effects. This relationship can be explained by the influence of hydrophobicity on the interaction of local anesthetics with neuronal and cardiac ion channels (see below).

Apart from lipophilic properties, local anesthetics differences in the clinical potency may be related to a number of other factors, such as molecular charge, vasodilator or vasoconstrictor properties, and the dosage of the local anesthetic [4]. As the dosage of an individual local anesthetic is increased, the onset of block becomes faster and the duration of analgesia increases. The dose of a local anesthetic can be increased by administering either a larger volume of the same concentration or by administering a more concentrated solution of the same volume. For example, increasing the concentration of bupivacaine from 0.125% to 0.5% without changing the injected volume results in shorter onset of action and a longer duration of analgesia but also in less differential nerve block (see below). The choice of the local anesthetic agent, the concentration of the chosen local anesthetic, and the volume injected together determine the clinical effect. In using local anesthetic agents for pain therapy, the desired analgesic effect has to be balanced against (1) the loss of differential nerve block (see below) and (2) the risk of adverse effects from excessive dosing or inadvertent systemic application. Table 6.2 provides a summary of pharmacological properties of local anesthetics.

Differential block of sensory and motor fibers

Therapy with local anesthetics aims at differentially blocking only those nerve fibers or nerve columns that carry undesired neurophysiological information

Table 6.2 Pharmacological Properties of Local Anesthetics

Agents	Molecular Weight	pK_a	Protein Binding (%)	Onset of Action	Duration of Action (h)	Potency
Esters						
Procaine	236	8.9	6	Long	1–1.5	0.5
Chloroprocaine	271	8.7	?	Short	0.5–1	1
Tetracaine	264	8.5	80	Long	3–4	4
Amides						
Lidocaine	234	7.9	65	Short	1.5–2	1
Prilocaine	220	7.6	55	Short	1.5–2	1
Mepivacaine	246	7.6	75	Short	2–3	1
Bupivacaine	288	8.1	95	Intermediate	3–3.5	4
Levobupivacaine	288	8.1	95	Intermediate	3–3.5	4
Etidocaine	276	7.7	95	Short	3–4	4
Ropivacaine	274	8.1	94	Intermediate	2.5–3	3.3

such as nociception. When a local anesthetic is used in a clinical setting, it is extremely helpful if the ascending nociceptive information is blocked without blockade of the descending motor information and hence without blocking motor neurons. The patients would then be free of pain but would still be capable of walking. Nerve fibers carrying sensory information are more susceptible to the pharmacological effects of local anesthetics than motor neurons [4]. Differential blockade of neural information can be achieved by the correct dosing of a local anesthetic. The higher the dose, the less differential the blockade of nerve fibers will be, and the more blockade of motor neurons will result.

Differential nerve block can be achieved with a wide variety of different local anesthetics because differential nerve block does not solely result from the pharmaceutical structure of a specific local anesthetic. Bupivacaine became popular in the 1980s for epidural blocks because it seemed better than the previously available long-acting agents (such as etidocaine) in producing adequate antinociception without profound inhibition of motor activity. Ropivacaine became popular in the 1990s and early 2000s for the same reason and was compared in several studies with bupivacaine. However, very rarely in these studies have equipotent solutions of study drugs been used [13].

Given the complex interaction of local anesthetic with tissue and nerves and the amount of confounding influence on local anesthetic drug effects, a more simplistic approach to the choice of drug may be warranted. Because achieving differential nerve block largely depends on the concentration and the injected volume of a given local anesthetic, the use of only two local anesthetics, mepivacaine and bupivacaine, allows the successful performance of several thousand peripheral nerve and central neuraxial blocks in our institution. Two additional local anesthetics, prilocaine and ropivacaine, were added to our pharmacy solely for practical reasons attributable to the drug formulation as delivered by the manufacturers.

Toxicity of local anesthetics

As a clinically applicable rule of thumb, it seems fair to assume that the higher the hydrophobicity or the higher the octanol-buffer coefficient, the slower the onset; however, the higher the potency, the longer the duration of effect, but also the higher the risk of severe side effects after inadvertent systemic application (Figure 6.1). Local anesthetics with a short or medium duration of action (such as lidocaine or mepivacaine) have a relatively wide therapeutic margin even allowing, as in the case of lidocaine, intravenous application. However, long-acting local anesthetics without the potential to induce severe side effects have yet to be developed for clinical application. Whether this will be achieved by alternative pharmacological strategies remains an important area of research [14, 15].

The potency of local anesthetic interaction with many different cellular structures such as ion channels correlates with their octanol-buffer coefficient [16, 17]. The most famous explanation for this relationship is provided by the guarded receptor hypothesis (Figure 6.2). This hypothesis [18] states that local anesthetics are capable of suppressing cardiac action potentials by blocking sodium channels following drug binding to a partially hydrophobic site on the channel when they are open. The drug molecules disappear from the sodium channel when they are closed. However, the time constant for disappearance or unblock is determined by the hydrophobicity. The more hydrophobic the drug is, the slower this drug disappears from the receptor and hence the longer the duration of action. This result usually is desirable for the blockade of pain transmission in peripheral nerves. However, it is entirely undesirable at other parts of the body such as the central nervous system or the heart, where blockade of ion channels and other molecular structures [19] may cause severe arrhythmia and sudden cardiac death [20].

From a therapeutic point of view, severe side effects of local anesthetics can be divided into two classes: class A and class B side effects. Class A side effects result from inadvertent systemic application of the drug that results in direct drug effects on the brain or the cardiovascular system. This usually happens in drug-induced seizure and cardiac arrhythmia. Class A side effects are most dangerous when resulting from long-acting local anesthetics such as bupivacaine; therapy is then extremely challenging and needs to be installed quickly. However, with the advent of lipid rescue therapy, the situation has changed considerably and successful treatment of severe intoxication has become easier [6].

Class B side effects results from direct toxic drug effects on central and peripheral nerves that result in transient radicular irritation, peripheral neuropathies, or cauda equina syndrome. These underlying toxic mechanisms include induction of inflammation and apoptosis of nerve cells [21, 22]. To some extent, class B side effects depend on the choice of drug (lidocaine 5%) and the regional anesthetic technique (spinal anesthesia) [23]. These side effects may last from days to persistent nerve damage without therapeutic options if they result from direct drug effects. To reduce the risk for these side

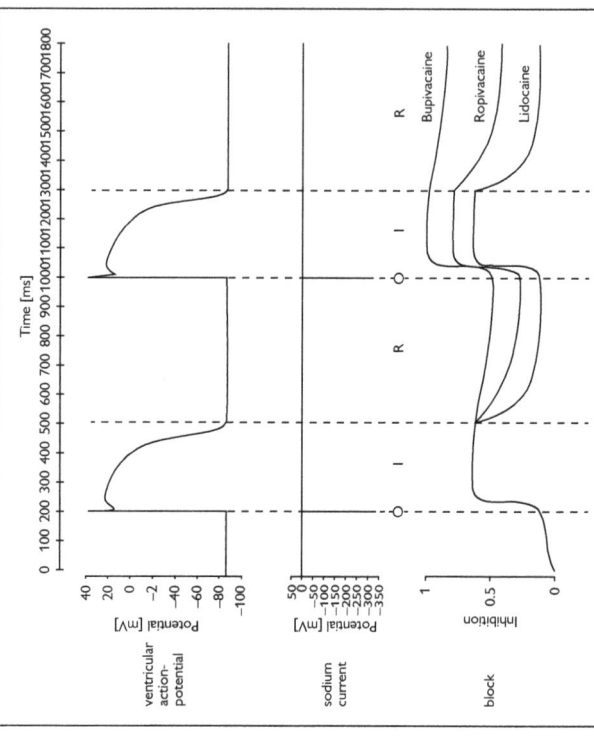

Figure 6.2 According to the guarded receptor hypothesis, local anesthetics block sodium currents during systole and dissociate from the ion channels during diastole. The time constant for disappearance is determined by the hydrophobicity. The more hydrophobic the drug, the slower this drug disappears from the channel and the higher the risk of cumulative block and cardiac arrhythmia. Experimental data on ropivacaine are limited. I, inactivated channel; O, open channel; R, resting channel.

effects, the maximum daily dose of local anesthetic should not be exceeded. When various local anesthetics are used, the doses are additive (Table 6.3).

Several epidemiologic studies [24, 25] report incidences of nerve injury such as transient radicular irritation, cauda equina syndrome, as well as peripheral neuropathies ranging from 1 in 8000 to 1 in 6. Due to their specific interactions with cardiac ion channels, local anesthetics are capable of inducing severe arrhythmias and cardiac arrest. Although the overall incidence of toxic complications seems low, local anesthetic-induced toxicity is not evenly distributed among different regional anesthetic techniques. In adult patients, major nerve blocks requiring large doses of local anesthetics are associated with a seizure incidence of up to 2 in 1000. Although no such complication was observed in caudal anesthesia, the incidence of cardiac arrest is 6 times higher (1 in 1600) in spinal anesthesia than in epidural anesthesia or major nerve block. Transient radicular irritation occurs more frequently than any other toxic side effect of local anesthetics with a reported incidence of up to 30%. Fortunately, neurotoxic side effects causing longer-term neurologic impairment such as cauda equina syndrome are rare, occurring in 1 in 10 000 patients. In a recent study [1] on the incidence of local anesthetic systemic toxicity and postoperative neurologic symptoms resulting from ultrasound-guided peripheral regional anesthetic techniques, the incidence was 1.8% for postoperative neurologic symptoms lasting longer than 5 days and 0.9 for postoperative neurologic symptoms lasting longer than 6 months. The incidence for seizure was below 0.1%, and cardiac arrests were not observed in the study population of more than 12 600 patients.

Clinical signs of local anesthetics toxicity are mostly cardiovascular and neurological (Table 6.4). Allergic reactions are rare after administration of a local anesthetic, but local anesthetics solutions can contain conservation agents, such as methylparabene, which can cause allergic reactions.

Lipid rescue therapy

Several case reports and animal studies over the last 15 years strongly suggest that infusing a cheap commercially available lipid emulsion usually given for parenteral nutrition constitutes an excellent treatment option for local anesthetic intoxication. Several mechanisms have been suggested to explain the beneficial effect of infusing a lipid emulsion in the case of local anesthetic intoxication such as the "lipid sink" theory and direct effects on cardiac metabolism [6]. The therapeutic approach of lipid infusion has widely been recognized and has been included in guidelines and recommendations as issued by

Table 6.3 Maximum Daily Doses of Local Anesthetics	
Cocaine	3 mg/kg
Lidocaine	4.5 mg/kg (7 mg/kg if used with epinephrine/adrenaline)
Prilocaine	8 mg/kg
Bupivacaine	3 mg/kg
Levobupivacaine	3 mg/kg
Ropivacaine	3 mg/kg

Table 6.4 Clinical Signs of Local Anesthetics Toxicity

Cardiovascular
- Atrioventricular conduction disturbances
- Rhythm disturbances (mostly ventricular: tachycardia, fibrillation)
- Asystole with cardiac arrest
- Hypotension
- Syncope

Neurological
- Peribuccal paresthesias
- Tinnitus
- Metallic taste
- Headaches
- Visual or auditory disturbances
- Tremors
- Loss of consciousness
- Coma
- Seizures
- Respiratory arrest

the Association of Anaesthetists of Great Britain and Ireland, the American Society of Regional Anesthesia [26], and the American Heart Association. The Helsinki Declaration on Patient Safety in Anaesthesiology requires that every department of anesthesiology in Europe provide a protocol for the management of local anesthetic toxicity. Several of these protocols are available online. It is advisable to only use local anesthetics for pain therapy when circumstances have been established that allow immediate state of the art resuscitation in case of local anesthetic intoxication.

References

1. Sites BD, Taenzer AH, Herrick MD, et al. Incidence of local anesthetic systemic toxicity and postoperative neurologic symptoms associated with 12,668 ultrasound-guided nerve blocks: an analysis from a prospective clinical registry. Reg Anesth Pain Med 2012; 37:478–482.

2. Yaksh TL, Luo ZD. Anatomy of the pain processing system. In: Waldman SD ed, *Pain Management*. 1st ed. Philadelphia, PA: Saunders; 2007: pp. 11–20.

3. Wedel DJ, Horlocker TT. Nerve blocks. In: Miller R, ed. *Miller's Anesthesia*. 7th ed. Philadelphia, PA: Churchill Livingstone; 2010: pp. 1639–1674.

4. Berde CB, Strichartz GR. Local anesthetics. In: Miller R, ed. *Miller's Anesthesia*. 7th ed. Philadelphia, PA: Churchill Livingstone; 2010: pp. 913–939.

5. Gray A. Ultrasound guidance for regional anesthesia. In: Miller R, ed. *Miller's Anesthesia*. 7th ed. Philadelphia, PA: Churchill Livingstone; 2010: pp. 1675–1704.

6. Weinberg GL. Lipid emulsion infusion: resuscitation for local anesthetic and other drug overdose. Anesthesiology 2012; 117:180–187.

7. Herroeder S, Pecher S, Schönherr ME, et al. Systemic lidocaine shortens length of hospital stay after colorectal surgery: a double-blinded, randomized, placebo-controlled trial. Ann Surg 2007; 246:192–200.

8. Marret E, Rolin M, Beaussier M, Bonnet F. Meta-analysis of intravenous lidocaine and postoperative recovery after abdominal surgery. Br J Surg 2008; 95:1331–1338.

9. De Oliveira GS Jr, Fitzgerald P, Streicher LF, et al. Systemic lidocaine to improve postoperative quality of recovery after ambulatory laparoscopic surgery. Anesth Analg 2012; 115:262–267.

10. Chen WK, Miao CH. The effect of anesthetic technique on survival in human cancers: a meta-analysis of retrospective and prospective studies. PLoS One 2013; 8:e56540.

11. Piegeler T, Votta-Velis EG, Liu G, et al. Antimetastatic potential of amide-linked local anesthetics: inhibition of lung adenocarcinoma cell migration and inflammatory Src signaling independent of sodium channel blockade. Anesthesiology 2012; 117:548–559.

12. Stow PJ, Glynn CJ, Minor B. EMLA cream in the treatment of post herpetic neuralgia: efficacy and pharmacokinetic profile. Pain 1989; 39:301–305.

13. Attal N, Cruccu G, Baron R, et al. EFNS guidelines on the pharmacological treatment of neuropathic pain: 2010 revision. Eur J Neurol 2010; 17:1113-e88.

14. Polley LS, Columb MO. Ropivacaine and bupivacaine: concentrating on dosing! Anesth Analg 2003; 96:1251–1253.

15. Kohane DS, Smith SE, Louis DN, et al. Prolonged duration local anesthesia from tetrodotoxin-enhanced local anesthetic microspheres. Pain 2003; 104:415–421.

16. Weiniger CF, Golovanevski L, Domb AJ, Ickowicz D. Extended release formulations for local anaesthetic agents. Anaesthesia 2012; 67:906–916.

17. Punke MA, Friederich P. Lipophilic and stereospecific interactions of amino-amide local anesthetics with human Kv1.1 channels. Anesthesiology 2008; 109:895–904.

18. Siebrands CC, Friederich P. Structural requirements of human ether-a-go-go-related gene channels for block by bupivacaine. Anesthesiology 2007; 106:523–531.

19. Clarkson CW, Hondeghem LM. Mechanism for bupivacaine depression of cardiac conduction: fast block of sodium channels during the action potential with slow recovery from block during diastole. Anesthesiology 1985; 62:396–405.

20. Butterworth JF 4th. Models and mechanisms of local anesthetic cardiac toxicity: a review. Reg Anesth Pain Med 2010; 35:167–176.

21. Albright GA. Cardiac arrest following regional anesthesia with etidocaine or bupivacaine. Anesthesiology 1979; 51:285–287.

22. Friederich P, Schmitz TP. Lidocaine-induced cell death in a human model of neuronal apoptosis. Eur J Anaesthesiol 2002; 19:564–570.

23. Werdehausen R, Fazeli S, Braun S, et al. Apoptosis induction by different local anaesthetics in a neuroblastoma cell line. Br J Anaesth 2009; 103:711–718.

24. Zaric D, Pace NL. Transient neurologic symptoms (TNS) following spinal anaesthesia with lidocaine versus other local anaesthetics. Cochrane Database Syst Rev 2009 Apr 15;(2):CD003006.

25. Auroy Y, Narchi P, Messiah A, et al. Serious complications related to regional anesthesia: results of a prospective survey in France. Anesthesiology 1997; 87:479–486.

26. Auroy Y, Benhamou D, Bargues L, et al. Major complications of regional anesthesia in France: The SOS Regional Anesthesia Hotline Service. Anesthesiology 2002; 97:1274–1280.

Chapter 7

N-Methyl-D-aspartate Antagonists

Philippe Richebé, Laurent Bollag, and Cyril Rivat

N-Methyl-D-aspartate (NMDA) receptor antagonists have been used in the field of perioperative pain management not for their direct analgesic effects but for their ability to reduce postoperative central pain sensitization and its clinical symptoms such as hyperalgesia, allodynia, and the development of chronic postsurgical pain. The use of NMDA receptor antagonists for chronic neuropathic pain has been less studied. Nevertheless, in this chapter, we will review their effect on both acute postoperative pain and chronic pain conditions.

To better understand the role of NMDA receptor antagonists and to introduce what is expected from their use in the clinical setting, it is important to define the clinical signs of pain hypersensitivity, namely allodynia and hyperalgesia.

The definition of hyperalgesia and allodynia

Acute intraoperative and postoperative pain is known to induce peripheral and central pain sensitization, similarly to what is seen in chronic pain conditions. The clinical symptoms encountered are called allodynia and hyperalgesia. Allodynia is defined by the International Association for the Study of Pain as "pain due to a stimulus that does not normally provoke pain." In the perioperative field, it might be defined as a nonpainful mechanical stimulation that becomes painful after tissue injury. Hyperalgesia is referred to as a mechanical stimulation that is slightly painful and becomes much more painful after tissue injury. Indirect markers of pain hypersensitivity are pain scores at rest and/or on movement and analgesic consumption (opioid titration, patient-controlled analgesia, or rescue analgesia use).

It is possible to differentiate between peripheral and central sensitization in the clinical setting. In the context of postoperative pain, peripheral sensitization is correlated with hypersensitivity generated at the peripheral nerve level, and it can be evaluated by mechanical stimulations next to the wound, 1–2 cm apart [1]. This phenomenon is called "primary hyperalgesia." Central sensitization occurs at the central nervous system level (spinal and supra-spinal level) and is evaluated further away from the wound, beyond the immediate area of inflammation. The area of hyperalgesia is then measured and an index can be calculated [2, 3]. More complex tools have also been reported to evaluate this central sensitization (RIII reflex etc…) [4, 5]. Some authors developed further experimental models in human volunteers in order to evaluate the therapeutic impact of so-called anti-hyperalgesic drugs [6, 7].

The consequences of postoperative hyperalgesia

After surgery, patients with a high level of hyperalgesia will likely experience:

- Increased postoperative pain and increased analgesic consumption

An association between hyperalgesia/allodynia and higher postoperative pain scores has been reported in some clinical trials, although conflicting results have been reported. In randomized controlled trials (RCTs) in which subjects were instructed to use patient-controlled analgesia (PCA) providing pain intensity of 4/10 or less, the most hypersensitive patients had higher opioid requests and consumption [2].

- Increased likelihood of long-term chronic pain

Long-term postoperative pain has been reported in many studies [8, 9], and its occurrence is correlated with acute postoperative hyperalgesia [3, 10, 11]. Long-term residual postoperative pain is often described as a neuropathic-like pain [9].

The key receptors involved in the activation of central pain sensitization process are the glutamate receptors, such as NMDA receptors. N-Methyl-D-aspartate receptors are activated when high intensity of painful stimulation occurs as seen during and after surgery. High doses of opioids given during and after surgery have also been shown to activate NMDA receptors and, as a consequence, to induce higher level of central pain sensitization and postoperative hyperalgesia, which in turn increases the risk of developing chronic pain.

Therefore, NMDA receptors modulation and/or blockade might be an interesting perioperative strategy to reduce central pain sensitization and to improve pain management intra- and postoperatively.

N-methyl-D-aspartate modulators as adjuvants of postoperative pain management

Intraoperative opioid management

There is considerable evidence, from both animal and clinical studies, that high intraoperative doses of opioids might increase postoperative central pain sensitization, hyperalgesia, and allodynia. Decreasing the total amount of opioid used during anesthesia helps with postoperative pain management and decreases postoperative hyperalgesia, allodynia, pain intensity, and opioid consumption [2, 12–14]. This is true for all types of opioids used during anesthesia and given by all routes of administration [2, 13].

Even if opioids are not per se drugs that have a direct effect on NMDA receptors, it has been reported that the activation of μ-opioid receptors indirectly phosphorylates and then modulates NMDA receptors' function. This hypothesis explains why high intraoperative doses of opioids induce the so-called "Opioid Induced Hyperalgesia (OIH)" [15, 16] (Figure 7.1).

"Reduction of high intraoperative doses of opioids" is therefore proposed as a beneficial strategy to decrease their effect on NMDA receptors activation and its consequence in terms of postoperative acute hyperalgesia and acute and chronic pain [17]. Other opioid-sparing techniques that reduce postoperative OIH include intraoperative regional anesthesia [18].

Ketamine

Ketamine is an NMDA-receptor antagonist. It blocks this receptor channel by acting on a specific subunit of the receptor. Plasma concentration of ketamine at 30 ng/mL seems to be sufficient to achieve a minimal analgesic effect [19] and to obtain a decrease in pain and opioid consumption after surgery [20, 21].

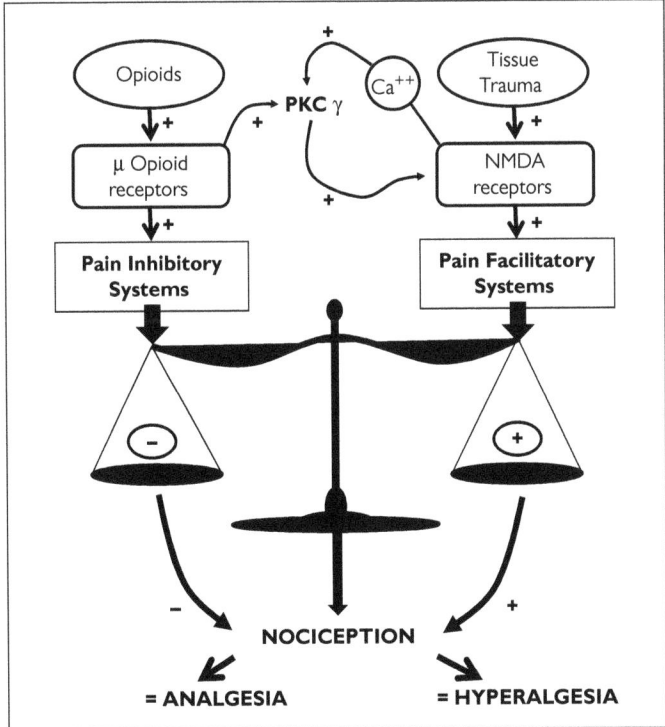

Figure 7.1 The graphic illustrates the link between μ-opioid receptors and N-methyl-D-aspartate (NMDA) receptors. By activating a specific protein kinase C γ, opioids have the ability to modulate or enhance the activity of NMDA receptors. This might lead to an exaggeration of postoperative hyperalgesia. Adapted from [16] with permission of Wolters Kluwer.

Administered during and after surgery, ketamine has been shown to reduce hyperalgesia when tested around the surgical wound [2, 22, 23].

Several recent meta-analyses demonstrated that the beneficial effect of ketamine on postoperative pain and opioid consumption was lasting beyond the elimination half-life of the drug [24–29]. These findings suggest that ketamine possesses a longer lasting effect than its own pharmacologic effect to block pain sensitization processes after surgery. As a consequence, ketamine demonstrated long-lasting effects on the development of long-term pain sensitization. The most recent meta-analysis to date indicated that a large majority of clinical trials favor the use of perioperative ketamine for acute pain management [27].

There is considerable variability of the ketamine regimens used in the literature to obtain an anti-hyperalgesic effect and to reduce acute postoperative pain and opioid requirements. Table 7.1 presents regimens that appear to be practical and relevant [27, 30]. Intra- and postoperative intravenous (i.v.) low doses of ketamine were also shown to reduce the development of chronic pain at 6 months or 12 months after laparotomies [3, 8, 31].

Finally, the epidural administration of ketamine was reported to effectively block pain sensitization [32]. However, this is not a recommended mode of usage, due to the possible neurotoxic effect of the various solutions used in different countries.

Other authors also reported on the use of S-ketamine. Regular ketamine is a racemic mixture of S(+) ketamine and R(−) ketamine. However, S(+) ketamine alone is now available in some countries. Its NMDA receptor affinity is four times greater than that of R(−) ketamine, and the analgesic effect is said to be 2–3 times greater than the racemic presentation of the drug. More clinical studies are needed to understand the role that S(+) ketamine will play in perioperative pain management.

Table 7.1 Recommendations for Intravenous Ketamine Use in Regards to the Level of Expected Postoperative Pain

			Surgery	
			Moderate Pain	**High Level of Pain**
Ketamine	Induction		0.25 mg/kg	0.5 mg/kg
	Maintenance	Repeated boluses (stop bolusing 30 min before end of surgery)	0.125 mg/kg every 30 min	0.25 mg/kg every 30 min
		Continuous infusion	0.25 mg/kg per h = 5 µg/kg per min	0.25 mg/kg per h = 5 µg/kg per min
	Postoperative		none	0.125 mg/kg per h = 2 µg/kg per min for 48 h

Ketamine has psychomimetic and hallucinogenic side effects mostly when used in anesthestic doses. However, some studies noted same side effects when only small subanesthetic doses were used [33, 34]. To minimize these side effects, it is recommended not to exceed intra- and postoperatively the above-mentioned subanesthetic ketamine doses.

The combination of ketamine with the solution of the opioid used in the PCA offered to the patient for managing his pain appeared inferior to a continuous infusion of ketamine separated from the i.v. opioid PCA. Therefore, the association ketamine/opioid in the same solution cannot be recommended [35, 36].

The future challenge will be to find the right patient population that will maximally benefit from perioperative ketamine utilization. Current meta-analyses in the literature are reporting a vast majority of RCTs in favor of ketamine improving postoperative pain management [27]. Unfortunately, these meta-analyses do not identify preoperative risk factors differentiating between high- and low-risk patients in terms of pain development and pain persistence. Nevertheless, it seems likely that a patient with a high preoperative risk for pain sensitization (for example, a patient with chronic pain condition and chronic opioid tolerance) would benefit more from ketamine administration than a low-risk patient. One recent study [39] demonstrated ketamine's beneficial effects on postoperative pain management in high-risk patients with chronic pain and chronic opioid exposure.

Because a patient is only once in his life "naive" in terms of pain sensitization, that is, before he undergoes his first "major surgery," we suggest that NMDA blockade or modulation should be given to everybody perioperatively. Future studies will have to address this issue and will evaluate whether ketamine should only be used in a specific, high-risk population or should be used for all patients.

Other *N*-methyl-D-aspartate antagonists and perioperative pain management

Memantine (NMDA receptor antagonist), amantadine (antiviral drug originally used to treat flu symptoms, antiparkinsonian drug; weak NMDA receptor antagonist effects), and methadone (μ-receptor opioid agonist and NMDA receptor antagonist) also antagonize NMDA receptors. Based on the very poor literature addressing the utilization of these drugs, no recommendation for clinical practice can be made to date in the perioperative setting.

Dextromethorphan has been proposed as an adjuvant for postoperative pain management also because of its anti-NMDA properties [38], but this drug has been abandoned and removed from the market in some European countries. Recommendation for its clinical use cannot be done based on the current literature.

Magnesium

Magnesium is the physiological NMDA receptor blocker, when the receptor is in its inactive state. As shown in a very recent and outstanding study, magnesium injected intravenously does not cross the blood-brain barrier [39].

Most animal studies using magnesium to block NMDA receptors reported outstanding results [40–43]. However, evidence from RCTs is conflicting, with some reporting positive results of i.v. magnesium to improve postoperative pain management [44–46], and others failing to support its use [47–49]. This lack of effect of i.v. magnesium might be explained by the poor crossing of the blood-brain barrier, as mentioned above. Nevertheless, a recent meta-analysis reported that i.v. magnesium given perioperatively could decrease the overall 24 hour morphine consumption by 24.4% and, to a lesser extent, postoperative pain intensity (4.2 at rest, 9.2 on movement on a scale of 100) [50]. In most studies, magnesium is administered as an i.v. bolus of 30–50 mg/kg at the time of anesthesia induction, and it is continued intra- and postoperatively with an average of 500 mg/h for 24 hours [50].

When given intrathecally or epidurally in humans, magnesium might have beneficial effect in perioperative pain management, but more studies are needed for this specific route of administration [3, 12, 55, 63]. Hemodynamic side effects might be of concern.

Nitrous Oxide

Nitrous oxide (N_2O) has been used in anesthesia for more than 150 years. It has sedative, analgesic, and anxiolytic properties. It is an NMDA receptor antagonist [55, 56]. Animal studies reported promising anti-hyperalgesic effect and an improvement of opioid tolerance in animals receiving N_2O only intraoperatively [57]. In humans, even if N_2O has been used in anesthesia for more than 150 years, no study has yet been designed to look at the impact of its intraoperative administration on postoperative pain, hyperalgesia, and opioid consumption. Future studies will have to address this question in clinical practice.

N-Methyl-D-aspartate modulators as adjuvants of chronic pain management

Ketamine is the NMDA receptor antagonist also used in the management of chronic pain. However, most chronic pain patients do not have i.v. access in the long term. As a consequence, low doses of i.v. ketamine are not the right strategy for chronic pain patients. Other routes of administration must be considered in this specific population.

A literature review evaluated 29 studies (579 patients) and suggested that ketamine might improve pain scores in patients with chronic noncancer pain. However, extended ketamine usage might be problematic due to lessened efficacy and poor tolerance [58]. One study showed a possible beneficial effect of ketamine in the treatment of complex regional pain syndrome [59]. Finally, ketamine is a "controlled-substance" in many countries, complicating patient access.

Given orally, ketamine has a bioavailability of 20% with an onset time of 30 minutes, whereas its bioavailability is 93% when given intramuscularly with an onset time of 5 minutes. Its analgesic effect duration is approximately 3 hours when given orally. Some authors suggested that oral ketamine might be even more potent than when given parenterally (ratio 3–2:1). When given by this route, dosing starts with 0.5 mg/kg orally with an increase of 0.5 mg/kg every 4 days to a maximum of 1000 mg per day.

In cancer pain, two articles concluded that there is not enough evidence to support the use of oral ketamine [60]. Ketamine is then used in selected patients, demonstrating either high opioid tolerance, resistance to opioids usage, or presenting intolerable opioid-related side effects [61].

Hence, despite the fact that many clinicians reported on the use of ketamine as an adjuvant medication in the treatment of chronic pain, reports of this practice are anecdotal and no clinical recommendations can be made. Prospective double-blind studies on ketamine advantages in patients with chronic pain conditions must be done on large populations in order to provide sufficient evidence on safety and efficacy, which will help to build robust recommendation to support ketamine use in chronic pain patients [58, 62, 63]. The same conclusion applies to the other NMDA modulators/antagonists mentioned in the previous section.

Conclusion

N-Methyl-D-aspartate receptor modulation has an important role in the management of postoperative pain. Ketamine is the most commonly used NMDA receptor antagonist by anesthesiologists and pain physicians to prevent postoperative central pain sensitization, to improve postoperative pain management, and perhaps to decrease long-term postoperative chronic pain. Other NMDA receptor modulators, for example magnesium or N_2O, require further evaluation in terms of their effects on postoperative pain.

Ketamine and other NMDA receptors could be administered orally for chronic pain conditions. However, further clinical studies need to look at toxicity, safety, and efficacy of ketamine (or any other NMDA antagonist) when administered for a prolonged period.

References

1. Albrecht E, Kirkham KR, Liu SS, Brull R. Peri-operative intravenous administration of magnesium sulphate and postoperative pain: a meta-analysis. Anaesthesia 2013; 68:79–90.

2. Angst MS, Clark JD. Opioid-induced hyperalgesia: a qualitative systematic review. Anesthesiology 2006; 104:570–587.

3. Arcioni R, Palmisani S, Tigano S, et al. Combined intrathecal and epidural magnesium sulfate supplementation of spinal anesthesia to reduce post-operative analgesic requirements: a prospective, randomized, double-blind, controlled trial in patients undergoing major orthopedic surgery. Acta Anaesthesiol Scand 2007; 51:482–489.

4. Azari P, Lindsay DR, Briones D, et al. Efficacy and safety of ketamine in patients with complex regional pain syndrome: a systematic review. CNS Drugs 2012; 26:215–228.

5. Begon S, Alloui A, Eschalier A, et al. Assessment of the relationship between hyperalgesia and peripheral inflammation in magnesium-deficient rats. Life Sci 2002; 70:1053–1063.

6. Begon S, Pickering G, Eschalier A, Dubray C. Magnesium and MK-801 have a similar effect in two experimental models of neuropathic pain. Brain Res 2000; 887:436–439.

7. Begon S, Pickering G, Eschalier A, Dubray C. Magnesium increases morphine analgesic effect in different experimental models of pain. Anesthesiology 2002; 96:627–632.

8. Begon S, Pickering G, Eschalier A, et al. Role of spinal NMDA receptors, protein kinase C and nitric oxide synthase in the hyperalgesia induced by magnesium deficiency in rats. Br J Pharmacol 2001; 134:1227–1236.

9. Bell RF. Ketamine for chronic non-cancer pain. Pain 2009; 141:210–214.

10. Bell RF, Dahl JB, Moore RA, Kalso E. Peri-operative ketamine for acute postoperative pain: a quantitative and qualitative systematic review (Cochrane review). Acta Anaesthesiol Scand 2005; 49:1405–1428.

11. Bilgin, H., B. Ozcan, et al. 2005; The influence of timing of systemic ketamine administration on postoperative morphine consumption. Journal of clinical anesthesia 17:592–597.

12. Bilir A, Gulec S, Erkan A, Ozcelik A. Epidural magnesium reduces postoperative analgesic requirement. Br J Anaesth 2007; 98:519–523.

13. Blonk MI, Koder BG, van den Bemt PM, Huygen FJ. Use of oral ketamine in chronic pain management: a review. Eur J Pain 2010; 14:466–472.

14. Bowdle TA, Radant AD, Cowley DS, et al. Psychedelic effects of ketamine in healthy volunteers: relationship to steady-state plasma concentrations. Anesthesiology 1998; 88:82–88.

15. Carstensen M, Moller AM. Adding ketamine to morphine for intravenous patient-controlled analgesia for acute postoperative pain: a qualitative review of randomized trials. Br J Anaesth 2010; 104:401–406.

16. Chauvin M, Fletcher D, Richebé P, French Society of Anesthesia and Resuscitation. [How can we use antihyperalgesic drugs?] Ann Fr Anesth Reanim 2009; 28:e13–25.

17. Chia YY, Liu K, Wang JJ, et al. Intraoperative high dose fentanyl induces postoperative fentanyl tolerance. Can J Anaesth 1999; 46:872–877.

18. Clements JA, Nimmo WS. Pharmacokinetics and analgesic effect of ketamine in man. Br J Anaesth 1981; 53:27–30.

19. De Kock M, Lavand'homme P, Waterloos H. 'Balanced analgesia' in the peri-operative period: is there a place for ketamine? Pain 2001; 92:373–380.

20. Dirks J, Moiniche S, Hilsted KL, Dahl JB. Mechanisms of postoperative pain: clinical indications for a contribution of central neuronal sensitization. Anesthesiology 2002; 97:1591–1596.

21. Duedahl TH, Romsing J, Møiniche S, Dahl JB. A qualitative systematic review of peri-operative dextromethorphan in post-operative pain. Acta Anaesthesiol Scand 2006; 50:1–13.

22. Eisenach JC. Preventing chronic pain after surgery: who, how, and when? Reg Anesth Pain Med 2006; 31:1–3.

23. Elia N, Tramer MR. Ketamine and postoperative pain—a quantitative systematic review of randomised trials. Pain 2005; 113:61–70.

24. Guignard B, Bossard AE, Coste C, et al. Acute opioid tolerance: intraoperative remifentanil increases postoperative pain and morphine requirement. Anesthesiology 2000; 93:409–417.

25. Guirimand F, Dupont X, Brasseur L, et al. The effects of ketamine on the temporal summation (wind-up) of the R(III) nociceptive flexion reflex and pain in humans. Anesth Analg 2000; 90:408–414.

26. Himmelseher S, Durieux ME. Ketamine for perioperative pain management. Anesthesiology 2005; 102:211–220.

27. Hood DD, Curry R, Eisenach JC. Intravenous remifentanil produces withdrawal hyperalgesia in volunteers with capsaicin-induced hyperalgesia. Anesth Analg 2003; 97:810–815.

28. Jevtovic-Todorovic V, Todorovic SM, Mennerick S, et al. Nitrous oxide (laughing gas) is an NMDA antagonist, neuroprotectant and neurotoxin. Nat Med 1998; 4:460–463.

29. Joly V, Richebe P, Guignard B, et al. Remifentanil-induced postoperative hyperalgesia and its prevention with small-dose ketamine. Anesthesiology 2005; 103:147–155.

30. Kehlet H, Jensen TS, Woolf CJ. Persistent postsurgical pain: risk factors and prevention. Lancet 2006; 367:1618–1625.

31. Koppert W, Dern SK, Sittl R, et al. A new model of electrically evoked pain and hyperalgesia in human skin: the effects of intravenous alfentanil, S(+)-ketamine, and lidocaine. Anesthesiology 2001; 95:395–402.

32. Laskowski K, Stirling A, McKay WP, Lim HJ. A systematic review of intravenous ketamine for postoperative analgesia. Can J Anaesth 2011; 58:911–923.

33. Lavand'homme P. Perioperative pain. Curr Opin Anaesthesiol 2006; 19:556–561.

34. Lavand'homme P, De Kock M, Waterloos H. Intraoperative epidural analgesia combined with ketamine provides effective preventive analgesia in patients undergoing major digestive surgery. Anesthesiology 2005; 103:813–820.

35. Lin SL, Tsai RY, Shen CH, et al. Co-administration of ultra-low dose naloxone attenuates morphine tolerance in rats via attenuation of NMDA receptor neurotransmission and suppression of neuroinflammation in the spinal cords. Pharmacol Biochem Behav 2010; 96:236–245.

36. Loftus RW, Yeager MP, Clark JA, et al. Intraoperative ketamine reduces perioperative opiate consumption in opiate-dependent patients with chronic back pain undergoing back surgery. Anesthesiology 2010; 113:639–646.

37. Lysakowski C, Dumont L, Czarnetzki C, Tramèr MR. Magnesium as an adjuvant to postoperative analgesia: a systematic review of randomized trials. Anesth Analg 2007; 104:1532–1539, table of contents.

38. Martinez, V., D. Fletcher, et al. 2007; The evolution of primary hyperalgesia in orthopedic surgery: quantitative sensory testing and clinical evaluation before and after total knee arthroplasty. Anesth Analg 105:815–821.

39. McCartney CJ, Sinha A, Katz J. A qualitative systematic review of the role of N-methyl-d-aspartate receptor antagonists in preventive analgesia. Anesth Analg 2004; 98:1385–1400, table of contents.

40. Meleine MC, Rivat C, Laboureyras E, et al. Sciatic nerve block fails in preventing the development of late stress-induced hyperalgesia when high-dose fentanyl is administered perioperatively in rats. Reg Anesth Pain Med 2012; 37:448–454.

41. Mercieri M, De Blasi RA, Palmisani S, et al. Changes in cerebrospinal fluid magnesium levels in patients undergoing spinal anaesthesia for hip arthroplasty: does intravenous infusion of magnesium sulphate make any difference? A prospective, randomized, controlled study. Br J Anaesth 2012; 109:208–215.

42. Mikkelsen S, Dirks J, Fabricius P, et al. Effect of intravenous magnesium on pain and secondary hyperalgesia associated with the heat/capsaicin sensitization model in healthy volunteers. Br J Anaesth 2001; 86:871–873.

43. Mion G, Tourtier JP, Rousseau JM. Ketamine in PCA: what is the effective dose? Eur J Anaesthesiol 2008; 25:1040–1041.

44. Noppers I, Niesters M, Aarts L, et al. Ketamine for the treatment of chronic non-cancer pain. Expert Opin Pharmacother 2010; 11:2417–2429.

45. Owen H, Reekie RM, Clements JA, et al. Analgesia from morphine and ketamine. A comparison of infusions of morphine and ketamine for postoperative analgesia. Anaesthesia 1987; 42:1051–1056.

46. Ozyalcin NS, Yucel A, Camlica H, et al. Effect of pre-emptive ketamine on sensory changes and postoperative pain after thoracotomy: comparison of epidural and intramuscular routes. Br J Anaesth 2004; 93:356–361.

47. Quibell R, Prommer EE, Mihalyo M, et al. Ketamine*. J Pain Symptom Manage 2011; 41:640–649.

48. Quinlan J. The use of a subanesthetic infusion of intravenous ketamine to allow withdrawal of medically prescribed opioids in people with chronic pain, opioid tolerance and hyperalgesia: outcome at 6 months. Pain Med 2012; 13:1524–1525.

49. Ranft A, Kurz J, Becker K, et al. Nitrous oxide (N2O) pre- and postsynaptically attenuates NMDA receptor-mediated neurotransmission in the amygdala. Neuropharmacology 2007; 52:716–723.

50. Richebe P, Rivat C, Creton C, et al. Nitrous oxide revisited: evidence for potent antihyperalgesic properties. Anesthesiology 2005; 103:845–854.

51. Schmid RL, Sandler AN, Katz J. Use and efficacy of low-dose ketamine in the management of acute postoperative pain: a review of current techniques and outcomes. Pain 1999; 82:111–125.

52. Simonnet G, Rivat C. Opioid-induced hyperalgesia: abnormal or normal pain? Neuroreport 2003; 14:1–7.

53. Steinlechner B, Dworschak M, Birkenberg B, et al. Magnesium moderately decreases remifentanil dosage required for pain management after cardiac surgery. Br J Anaesth 2006; 96:444–449.

54. Stubhaug A, Breivik H, Eide PK, et al. Mapping of punctuate hyperalgesia around a surgical incision demonstrates that ketamine is a powerful suppressor of central sensitization to pain following surgery. Acta Anaesthesiol Scand 1997; 41:1124–1132.

55. Sun J, Wu X, Xu X, et al. A comparison of epidural magnesium and/or morphine with bupivacaine for postoperative analgesia after cesarean section. Int J Obstet Anesth 2012; 21:310–316.

56. Suzuki M, Haraguti S, Sugimoto K, et al. Low-dose intravenous ketamine potentiates epidural analgesia after thoracotomy. Anesthesiology 2006; 105:111–119.

57. Suzuki M, Kinoshita T, Kikutani T, et al. Determining the plasma concentration of ketamine that enhances epidural bupivacaine-and-morphine-induced analgesia. Anesth Analg 2005; 101:777–784.

58. Tauzin-Fin P, Sesay M, Delort-Laval S, et al. Intravenous magnesium sulphate decreases postoperative tramadol requirement after radical prostatectomy. Eur J Anaesth 2006; 23:1055–1059.

59. Tramer MR, Glynn CJ. An evaluation of a single dose of magnesium to supplement analgesia after ambulatory surgery: randomized controlled trial. Anesth Analg 2007; 104:1374–1379, table of contents.

60. van Gulik L, Ahlers SJ, van de Garde EM, et al. Remifentanil during cardiac surgery is associated with chronic thoracic pain 1 yr after sternotomy. 2012; Br J Anaesth 109:616–622.
61. Webb AR, Skinner BS, Leong S, et al. The addition of a small-dose ketamine infusion to tramadol for postoperative analgesia: a double-blinded, placebo-controlled, randomized trial after abdominal surgery. Anesth Analg 2007; 104:912–917.
62. Wilder-Smith CH, Knopfli R, Wilder-Smith OH. Perioperative magnesium infusion and postoperative pain. Acta Anaesthesiol Scand 1997; 41:1023–1027.
63. Yousef AA, Amr YM. The effect of adding magnesium sulphate to epidural bupivacaine and fentanyl in elective caesarean section using combined spinal-epidural anaesthesia: a prospective double blind randomised study. Int J Obstet Anesth 2010; 19:401–404.

Chapter 8

Topical Adjuvant Analgesics

Jana Sawynok

Introduction

Topical analgesics represent a class of drugs that are applied to the skin and influence pain by local actions on sensory nerve endings and/or cellular targets adjacent to, and interacting with, such sensory nerve endings. They encompass such formulations as creams, lotions, gels, and sprays, as well as patches or plasters where the drug is embedded in a physical matrix. Some analgesics applied as a patch have systemic actions that influence pain signaling (eg, fentanyl), and are not regarded as topical analgesics. There are several advantages to the use of topical analgesics including low systemic drug levels, fewer systemic adverse effects (AEs), fewer drug interactions, and avoidance of factors that limit oral bioavailability (eg, first-pass metabolism). Limitations to this approach include access to site of action (the drug needs physicochemical properties that allow for dermal and tissue penetration), alteration of absorption by disease states of the skin, and local AEs in response to the drug (eg, redness, itching). Topical analgesics can be used either as single therapies or as adjuvants in combination with oral analgesics. In the latter instance, this would potentially allow for recruitment of multiple actions for suppressing pain without increasing the burden of systemic AEs. Topical analgesics may be of particular benefit in the elderly, where there are likely other medical conditions being treated with drugs (ie, polypharmacy is common), and avoidance of central nervous system effects (eg, sedation, confusion) is desirable.

Over the past decades, several topical analgesic formulations have been approved for use, and these include topical nonsteroidal anti-inflammatory drugs (NSAIDs) for inflammatory indications, topical local anesthetics as a plaster or patch for neuropathic pain, and, more recently, a high-concentration capsaicin patch for neuropathic pain. There is now a considerable body of evidence that indicates topical agents are indeed efficacious in these pain conditions when compared with placebo. More importantly, some studies also provide comparative data between topical and oral analgesics, as well as information on combinations of oral and topical analgesics. Taken together, this body of information provides validation for the approach of applying drugs locally to a site of action for pain relief in several pain conditions. The past decade has also seen identification of molecular mechanisms involved in peripheral pain signaling in neurons, as well as an increased understanding of the complexity of peripheral pain signaling mechanisms with interactions between neurons and adjacent structures, and there is considerable preclinical interest in the idea of developing novel topical analgesics. It is very likely that in the future, novel topical analgesics consisting of new molecular targets, as well as combinations of agents, will be developed, and these will provide clinicians with a greater range of therapeutic choices for pain management. This chapter will consider some key recent observations that validate and sustain an interest in this approach to pain management. Reference to a much more extensive body of literature can be found within cited reports.

Topical nonsteroidal anti-inflammatory drugs and pain

Earlier trials on topical NSAIDs were confounded by use of a heterogenous number of NSAID agents, trials of shorter duration, and mixed disease conditions. In the past decade, a coherent body of information on a single agent in more homogenous pain conditions, and for longer intervals (for 6–12 weeks), has been elaborated, and based on these findings, three topical NSAID formulations have been approved for use in the United States. Drugs approved by the US Food and Drug Administration (FDA) are diclofenac as a patch (1.3% epolamine salt, approved in 2007), as a gel (diclofenac sodium 1% gel [DSG], approved in 2007), and as a solution with dimethyl sulfoxide (DMSO) (1.5% sodium salt in 45.5% DMSO solution [D-DMSO], approved in 2009) [1]. The diclofenac epolamine patch is indicated for acute pain (strains, sprains, contusions), whereas the other two formulations are approved for treatment of osteoarthritis (OA) [1]. Diclofenac is a nonselective cyclo-oxygenase inhibitor, which leads to decreased production of proinflammatory prostaglandins that act on G-protein-coupled receptors on sensory nerve endings to sensitize sensory afferent neurons. Additional novel mechanisms (eg, block of N-methyl-D-aspartate receptors) may also be involved, especially when local tissue drug concentrations may be higher than those attained after systemic drug delivery.

Table 8.1 summarizes recent randomized controlled trials examining the efficacy of topical NSAIDs in OA. Two trials report reduced pain and improved physical function with topical DSG, compared with vehicle, with hand [2] and knee OA [3] over 8–12 weeks. Another trial reported improved pain and physical function with topical D-DMSO compared with vehicle with knee OA over 12 weeks [4]. The latter trial also compared topical D-DMSO with oral diclofenac and observed no difference in efficacy between the topical and oral formulations. It also included a combination topical diclofenac/oral diclofenac group and found that the combination had comparable efficacy to oral or topical diclofenac alone [4]. This result suggests either that addition of a topical agent with the same mechanism of action cannot augment the analgesia provided by the oral drug or that additivity can be difficult to demonstrate in this condition. Several of these trials share common characteristics, and they are amenable to pooled analysis. A pooled safety analysis of two trials indicates significantly more local skin AEs with the topical,

Table 8.1 Summary of Recent Randomized Controlled Trials of Topical NSAIDs for Osteoarthritis

Trial	Study Characteristics	Efficacy Outcomes	Safety Outcomes
Diclofenac Sodium Gel 1%			
Altman et al [2]	RCT hand OA	+OA pain	Local AEs
	DSG 4 × daily;	+AUSCAN	2.5% DSG vs 1.1% Veh
	vehicle	−Global	GI AEs
	8 weeks (N = 385)		7.6% DSG vs 3.7% Veh
Barthel et al [3]	RCT knee OA	+WOMAC pain	Local AEs
	DSG 4 × daily;	+ WOMAC function	5.1% DSG vs 2.5% Veh
	vehicle	+Global	GI AEs
	12 weeks (N = 492)		5.9% DSG vs 5.0% Veh
Diclofenac 1.5%/DMSO 45.5%			
Simon et al [4]	RCT knee OA	+WOMAC pain	Local AEs
	tDiclo 4 × daily;	+WOMAC function	26.6% tDiclo vs 7.6% P
	Placebo; DMSO;	+Global	vs 16.8% DMSO vs
	oDiclo; tDiclo/oDiclo		7.3% oDiclo vs 30.9% tDiclo/oDiclo
	12 weeks (N = 775)		
			GI AEs
			6.5% tDiclo vs 9.6% P vs 11.2% DMSO vs 23.8% oDiclo vs 25.7% tDiclo/oDiclo

AEs, adverse effects; AUSCAN, Australian/Canadian Osteoarthritis Hand Index; DMSO, dimethylsulfoxide; DSG, diclofenac sodium gel; GI, gastrointestinal; OA, osteoarthritis; oDiclo, oral diclofenac; P, placebo; RCT, randomized controlled trial; tDiclo, topical diclofenac; Veh, vehicle; WOMAC, Western Ontario and McMaster Universities Osteoarthritis Index.

compared with the oral, diclofenac (24.1% vs 1.9%) and fewer gastrointestinal AEs (25.4% vs 39.0%) but comparable cardiovascular AEs (1.5% vs 3.5%) [5]. A comparison of DSG effects in older (≥65 years) versus younger patients (<65 years) in a pooled analysis of three 12-week trials reported similar efficacy in both groups (improvements of 39%–46% compared with 28%–35% with placebo in younger patients vs 45%–50% compared with 35%–39% with placebo in older patients) [6]. Pooled safety analysis also indicated a similar profile in the two groups [6]. Meta-analysis of a larger and more heterogenous data set of topical NSAID drugs in older adults with OA reported up to 39.5% application-site AEs and 17.5% systemic AEs; conclusions of this meta-analysis suggest further data are required to determine safety of topical NSAIDs in the elderly [7].

Osteoarthritis is a chronic condition, and treatment guidelines emphasize the need for low-risk strategies. The above emerging body of information is recent, and it has not yet fully been incorporated into treatment guidelines. It indicates considerable promise for topical NSAIDs as a useful and safer treatment strategy for OA. For acute and chronic low back pain, widespread musculoskeletal pain, and peripheral neuropathic pain conditions, the current evidence does not support use of topical NSAIDs as analgesics [8].

Topical lidocaine and neuropathic pain

Lidocaine 5%, as a medicated plaster or patch (5% LMP), has been available in the United States for treatment of postherpetic neuralgia (PHN) since 1999, and is also currently available in Europe. The plaster is a 10 × 14 cm adhesive containing 700 mg (5% w/w) of lidocaine, and up to 3 patches are applied for up to 12 hours [9]. Lidocaine is a local anesthetic and is understood to act by inhibiting sodium channel activity; this results in reduced hyperactivity and reduced ectopic discharges in sensory afferent neurons. In human volunteers, acute patch application for 6 hours leads to inhibition of activity in small Aδ- and C-fibers, although the extent of block is variable [10]. In PHN patients, both acute (6 hours) and chronic (2 weeks) application of 5% LMP inhibits spontaneous pain, and this is reflected in reduced activity in several brain regions representing sensory, affective, and hedonic functions [11]. Pharmacokinetic studies indicate low systemic levels of lidocaine following patch application, with peak plasma concentrations after 14 hours and steady-state concentrations within 4 days [9].

The efficacy of 5% LMP in relieving pain in PHN, both compared with placebo and with other interventions, has been systematically reviewed recently [12]. Placebo-controlled studies indicate 5% LMP provides pain relief and reduces allodynia, with generally low AEs [12]. In addition, comparison of 5% LMP with pregabalin indicates noninferiority of the LMP with respect to pain relief, greater improvement in quality of life, and fewer AEs compared with oral pregabalin [12]. In a network meta-analysis for PHN studies, LMP and gabapentin differed from placebo; from another perspective, LMP had more effect than capsaicin, gabapentin, and pregabalin [12]. A systematic review of LMP for diabetic peripheral neuropathy (DPN) reported noninferiority to oral pregabalin with respect to pain reduction and fewer AEs [13]. Network meta-analysis for this condition showed all interventions (LMP, amitriptyline, capsaicin, gabapentin, pregabalin) differed from placebo [13]. In clinical practice, LMP has a favorable efficacy profile against neuropathic pain of mixed etiology (PHN, postsurgical, and posttraumatic neuropathic pain) with pain reductions of more than 50% in 45.5% and more than 30% in 82.2% of cases [14]. The lidocaine patch is now considered a first-line therapy for PHN, especially in elderly patients, and is most useful when the pain is well localized [15].

There are some data on combinations of 5% LMP with oral therapies for neuropathic pain. Thus, in those with PHN and painful DPN who fail to respond to either LMP or pregabalin as individual agents over 4 weeks, combination of the two approaches provides clinically relevant pain relief during the 8 week combination phase [16]. This treatment supports the general notion that addition of a topical regime to an oral regime, in which the two treatments have a different mechanism of action, can lead to enhanced analgesia. However, this approach will need to be evaluated in a prospective manner with combinations compared directly with monotherapy alone, and over a longer time interval. Given the limited efficacy of individual agents in treating neuropathic pain, there is increasing attention being given to combination therapies [17]. This approach is particularly amenable to topical therapies being added to oral therapies because of the relatively benign systemic side-effect profile of topical agents.

Topical capsaicin and neuropathic pain

Capsaicin is derived from hot chili peppers and has a long history of use in medical practice. Capsaicin interacts with transient receptor potential vanilloid 1 (TRPV1) receptors located on Aδ- and C-fibers, and it leads to cation entry into sensory afferents; chronic exposure to capsaicin desensitizes the channels, leads to loss of sensory integration, and results in analgesia. Topical low concentration capsaicin creams and patches (0.025%–0.1%, for daily use) have been available since the early 1980s and have been used to treat inflammatory (OA, rheumatoid arthritis) and neuropathic (PHN, DPN) pain conditions. The most recent meta-evaluation of efficacy of capsaicin 0.075% for neuropathic pain indicates efficacy is modest (number-needed-to-treat values of 6.6) and side effects (burning and stinging) are common (number-needed-to-harm values of 2.5) [18]. It was concluded that capsaicin cream, either alone or in combination with other agents, may be useful in those who do not respond to, or cannot tolerate, other treatments [18].

A high concentration (8%) capsaicin patch (Quetenza) was recently approved in 2009 in the European Union and the United States [19]. The patch is 280 cm^2, contains 179 mg of capsaicin (8% w/w), and is cut to match the size and shape of the painful area. At this concentration, the action of capsaicin is attributed to "defunctionalization" of nociceptors, which reflects loss of membrane potential, altered transport of neurotrophic factors, and reversible retraction of epidermal and dermal nerve fibers [9]. The 8% patch is usually compared with a 0.04% patch as the control condition, and the low concentration is sufficient to produce local reactions and blinding of the study treatment; whether the 0.04% patch also produces some analgesia cannot be determined from these studies. The 8% patch is generally applied for 60 minutes after application of topical local anesthetics (4% lidocaine or 2.5% prilocaine/2.5% lidocaine) to mitigate local pain reactions [20]. Application site pain can be further managed with oral analgesics and/or cooling (ice). Phase 3 studies (double-blind, multicentre trials) demonstrate a significant reduction in pain over 12 weeks in PHN and human immunodeficiency virus-associated neuropathy, with pain reductions of 30%–33% compared with 20%–25% in the control condition [19]. A comparison of 30-, 60-, and 90-minute patch applications in PHN indicates the longer times produced significant treatment effects [21]. In an open-label trial comparing outcomes in PHN and DPN, reductions in pain of 31% and 28% were observed over 2–12 weeks in these two groups, and there was a 47% and 44% responder rate (more than 30% reduction), respectively [22].

Pooled tolerability data from 8 randomized-controlled trials (N = 1327 participants) are available [23]. After patch application, 67% of participants report treatment-related AEs, which are most commonly application site reactions (erythema, pain); these resolve within 7 days. Rescue medication is higher after the 8% patch than for the control patch (0.04%). The incidence of AEs did not increase with multiple doses for up to 52 weeks (4 cycles). Sensory testing indicated that there was no evidence of impaired neurological function with respect to allodynia, sensations of warmth, vibration or pinprick, and deep tendon reflexes after patch application.

The question of whether the 8% capsaicin patch produces additive effects in combination with oral medications has been approached indirectly by analysis of integrated data from four controlled PHN studies [24]. In these studies, the 8% patch was administered alone or together with systemic neuropathic pain medications; in both cases, pain was reduced regardless of systemic drug use. However, there was no evidence of an additive effect seen with the combination of the topical and systemic agent, despite the recruitment of different mechanisms by the two approaches.

Novel topical agents and future directions

The above sections have focused on topical formulations that have been approved for use by the FDA in recent years. Clinical trials with these formulations provide a body of information that supports the efficacy of peripheral applications of drugs and indicate a low systemic AE profile. Although there can be dermal reactions with the topical approach, these are generally well tolerated. There is increasing attention being given to combination therapies for neuropathic pain [17], and this can include oral and topical formulations. There are some data, using both direct and indirect approaches, that address the potential of combinations between topical and oral medications, but there is a need for systematic prospective studies of this nature. There is also a developing clinical literature on analgesia following topical application of drugs regarded as investigational agents (eg, glyceryl trinitrate, antidepressants, ketamine, clonidine, and several other centrally acting drugs) [25]. In addition, it is now appreciated that compounds such as camphor, menthol, and eucalyptol (as well as other compounds present in traditional herbal remedies) act on several members of the transient receptor potential family of receptors (eg, TRPV3, TRPV4, TRPM8, TRPA1) and may have further direct and more complex actions on sensory signaling [26]. Furthermore, with the recent appreciation that keratinocytes interact with sensory neurons, are altered in chronic pain, and express TRP receptors [27], it may be that topical analgesics are able to act on both neurons and on keratinocytes in producing their effects on sensory function. The potential for recruiting local peripheral mechanisms is likely to receive considerable attention in the future as a novel and adjuvant strategy for the management of pain.

References

1. Argoff CE. Recent developments in the treatment of osteoarthritis with NSAIDs. Curr Med Res Opin 2011; 27:1315–1327.

2. Altman RD, Dreiser RL, Fisher CL, et al. Diclofenac sodium gel in patients with primary hand osteoarthritis: a randomized, double-blind, placebo-controlled trial. J Rheumatol 2009; 36:1991–1999.

3. Barthel HR, Haselwood D, Longley S 3rd, et al. Randomized controlled trial of diclofenac sodium gel in knee osteoarthritis. Semin Arthritis Rheum 2009; 39:203–212.

4. Simon LS, Grierson LM, Naseer Z, et al. Efficacy and safety of topical diclofenac containing dimethyl sulfoxide (DMSO) compared with those of topical placebo, DMSO vehicle and oral diclofenac for knee osteoarthritis. Pain 2009; 143:238–245.

5. Roth SH, Fuller P. Diclofenac topical solution compared with oral diclofenac: a pooled safety analysis. J Pain Res 2011; 4:159–167.

6. Argoff CE, Gloth FM. Topical nonsteroidal anti-inflammatory drugs for management of osteoarthritis in long-term care patients. Ther Clin Risk Manag 2011; 7:393–399.

7. Makris UE, Kohlwer MJ, Fraenkel L. Adverse effects of topical nonsteroidal anti-inflammatory drugs in older adults with osteoarthritis: a systematic literature review. J Rheumatol 2010; 37:1–8.

8. Haroutiunian S, Drennan DA, Lipman AG. Topical NSAID therapy for musculoskeletal pain. Pain Med 2010; 11:535–549.

9. Garnock-Jones KP, Keating GM. Lidocaine 5% medicated plaster. A review of its use in postherpetic neuralgia. Drugs 2009; 69:2149–2165.

10. Krumova EK, Zeller M, Westermann A, et al. Lidocaine patch (5%) induces partial blockade of Aδ- and C-fibers to variable extent. Pain 2012; 153:273–280.

11. Geha PY, Baliki MN, Chialvo DR, et al. Brain activity for spontaneous pain of postherpetic neuralgia and its modulation by lidocaine patch therapy. Pain 2007; 128:88–100.

12. Wolff RF, Bala MM, Westwood M, et al. 5% Lidocaine-medicated plaster vs other relevant interventions and placebo for post-herpetic neuralgia (PHN): a systematic review. Acta Neurol Scand 2011; 123:295–309.

13. Wolff RF, Bala MM, Westwood M, et al. 5% Lidocaine medicated plaster in painful diabetic neuropathy (DPN): a systematic review. Swiss Med Wkly 2010; 140:297–306.

14. Delorme C, Navez ML, Legout V, et al. Treatment of neuropathic pain with 5% lidocaine-medicated plaster: five years of clinical experience. Pain Res Manag 2011; 16:259–263.

15. Dworkin RH, O'Conner AB, Audette J, et al. Recommendations for the pharmacological management of neuropathic pain: an overview and literature update. Mayo Clin Proc 2010; 85(Suppl):S3–S14.

16. Baron R, Mayoral V, Leijon G, et al. Efficacy and safety of combination therapy with 5% lidocaine medicated plaster and pregabalin in post-herpetic neuralgia and diabetic polyneuropathy. Curr Med Res Opin 2009; 25:1677–1687.

17. Vorobeychik Y, Gordin V, Mao J, Chen L. Combination therapy for neuropathic pain. A review of current evidence. CNS Drugs 2011; 25:1023–1034.

18. Derry S, Lloyd R, Moore RA, et al. Topical capsaicin for chronic neuropathic pain in adults. Cochrane Database Syst Rev 2009 Oct 7;(4):CD007393.

19. Anand P, Bley K. Topical capsaicin for pain management: therapeutic potential and mechanisms of action of the new high-concentration capsaicin 8% patch. Br J Anesth 2011; 107:490–502.

20. Webster LR, Nunez M, Trak MD, et al. Tolerability of NGX-4010, a capsaicin 8% dermal patch, following pretreatment with lidocaine 2.5%/prilocaine 2.5% cream in patients with post-herpetic neuralgia. BMC Anesthesiol 2011; doi:10.1186/1471-2253-11-25.

21. Webster LR, Malan TP, Tuchman MM, et al. A multi-centre, randomized, double-blind, controlled dose finding study of NGX-4010, a high-concentration capsaicin patch, for the treatment of postherpetic neuralgia. J Pain 2010; 11:972–982.

22. Webster LR, Peppin JF, Murphy FT, et al. Efficacy, safety and tolerability of NGX-4010, capsaicin 8% patch, in an open-label study of patients with peripheral neuropathic pain. Diabetes Res Clin Pract 2011; 93:187–197.

23. McCormack PL. Capsaicin dermal patch. In non-diabetic peripheral neuropathic pain. Drugs 2010; 70:1831–1842.

24. Irving GA, Backonja M, Rauckj R, et al. NGX-4010, a capsaicin 8% dermal patch, administered alone or in combination with systemic neuropathic pain medications, reduces pain in patients with postherpetic neuralgia. Clin J Pain 2012; 28:101–107.

25. Zur E. Topical treatment of neuropathic pain using compounded medications. Clin J Pain 2013; 30:73–91.

26. Premkumar LS, Abooj M. TRP channels and analgesia. Life Sciences 2013; 92:415–424.

27. Smith HS. Pain—Skin deep at times? Pain Physician 2009; 12:919–921.

Chapter 9.1

Neuropathic Pain

Nadine Attal

Introduction

Neuropathic pain (NP) may arise as a consequence of a lesion or disease affecting the somatosensory system NP [1]. Neuropathic pain is estimated to affect as much as 7% of the general population in some European countries [2]. Classic examples of NP include diabetic polyneuropathies, postherpetic neuralgia, trigeminal neuralgia, and central poststroke or spinal cord injury (SCI) pain. Traumatic or postsurgical neuropathies and painful radiculopathies are also common conditions in the general population [2].

Patients with NP generally exhibit "spontaneous" (or stimulus-independent) and "evoked" (or stimulus-dependent) components, which often coexist. Spontaneous NP may be continuous (eg, foot pain in diabetic neuropathy) or intermittent (eg, pain paroxysms in trigeminal neuralgia). In addition to temporal variations in pain intensity, individuals with NP often report varying pain qualities, such as burning, cold, sharp, and squeezing [3]. Intermittent NP, often referred to as pain paroxysms, is often described as "shooting," "stabbing," or "electric shock-like" [4]. Evoked NP (hyperalgesia or allodynia) is generally defined with reference to the evoking stimulus and may be provoked by brush, pressure, cold, or heat [3]. More importantly, these neuropathic characteristics are shared by most NP etiologies, which indicates that despite obvious differences in etiology, the clinical entity of NP has strong clinical consistency [5].

Diagnosis of neuropathic pain

Several screening tools have been developed over the last 10 years for the identification of NP (refs in [6]). One feature common to all these tools is a reliance principally on verbal reports of pain qualities (ie, pain descriptors). Two of the five screening tools—the Leeds Assessment of Neuropathic Symptoms and Signs (LANSS) and the « Douleur Neuropathique en 4 questions » (DN4) questionnaires—are clinician-administered questionnaires including both items related to the interview (ie, symptoms) and items related to the sensory examination (ie, signs). The other three screening tools are self-administered questionnaires including only items related to the symptoms of NP: The Neuropathic Pain Questionnaire, ID Pain, and PainDetect.

Screening tools have gained acceptance in the medical community. Although these tools are based on descriptors, their linguistic adaptation and revalidation into different languages is feasible and ensures their reliability and validity in languages other than those in which they were initially developed. The major strength of these tools is to identify potential patients with NP, particularly by nonspecialists, but these tools have not been validated to measure NP symptoms for therapeutic intervention. The use of these tools in different languages and cultures should contribute to increase the recognition of NP, which is crucial for a better therapeutic management, and facilitate the conduct of badly needed epidemiology studies of NP in different countries. More importantly, however, screening tools fail to identify approximately 10%–20% of patients with clinician-diagnosed NP, indicating that they may offer guidance for further diagnostic evaluation and pain management but cannot replace clinical judgment.

Management of neuropathic pain

The management of patients with chronic NP is challenging [7–11], despite several attempts to develop a more rational therapeutic approach. Table 9.1.1 provides a detailed list of adjuvant analgesics recommended for use in neuropathic pain, along with mechanisms of action, dosing recommendations and most commonly reported adverse effects.

Peripheral neuropathic pain

Most studies of NP have been performed in postherpetic neuralgia (PHN) and diabetic painful polyneuropathy (PPN). These trials mainly studied the effects of monotherapy and were placebo controlled. Here, we will only focus on the drugs used at repeated dosages or topically; drugs used as intravenous injections will not be reviewed.

Tricyclic antidepressants

The efficacy of tricyclic antidepressants (TCAs) is established mainly in diabetic PPN and PHN. Their analgesic efficacy is independent of their antidepressant effect, and this efficacy is probably mediated by action on descending modulatory inhibitory controls, although a peripheral effect on sodium channels has also been reported [7, 9]. Tricyclic antidepressants should be initiated at low dosages (10–25 mg in a single dose at bedtime) and then slowly titrated as tolerated. The average dosage for amitriptyline is 75 mg/day, but effective dosages vary from one patient to another (eg, 25–150 mg of amitriptyline or equivalent). More information on various antidepressants used as adjuvant analgesics is provided in Chapter 3.

Serotonin-norepinephrine reuptake inhibitors

The efficacy of the serotonin-norepinephrine reuptake inhibitors (SNRIs) duloxetine and venlafaxine is established mainly in diabetic PPN [13]. However, recent studies have indicated that duloxetine has significant efficacy for other types of peripheral NP such as chemotherapy-induced neuropathy (see Chapter 9.2). Adequate dosages of duloxetine range between 60 and 120 mg/day, with no clear superiority of 120 mg. Treatment should be initiated at 30 mg/day to avoid nausea and then titrated to 60 mg/day after

Table 9.1.1 Summary of Evidence-Based Recommendations for Treatment of Peripheral Neuropathic Pain*

Drug	Main Mechanisms of Action	Common Major Side Effects	Precautions	Other Benefits	Efficacy; Level A/B Rating[a]	Starting Dose/ Maximum Dose	Titration
Tricyclic antidepressants							
Nortriptyline Desipramine Amitriptyline	Inhibition of reuptake of monoamines, block of sodium channels, anticholinergic	Somnolence, anticholinergic effects, weight gain	Cardiac disease (ECG), glaucoma, prostatic adenoma, seizure, use of tramadol	Improvement of depression, although at generally higher dosages than pain (75 mg/h) and sleep (amitriptyline)	A. Diabetic neuropathy, PHN B. Spinal cord injury/central poststroke pain, traumatic nerve lesions, cancer neuropathic pain	10–25 mg at bedtime/ 150 mg daily	Increase by 10 to 25 mg every 3 to 7 days up to efficacy and side effects
Serotonin–norepinephrine reuptake inhibitors							
Duloxetine	Inhibition of serotonin and norepinephrine reuptake	Nausea	Hepatic disorder, use of tramadol, hypertension	Improvement of depression and generalized anxiety, improvement of sleep	A. Diabetic neuropathy	30 mg once daily/60 mg twice daily	May start at 30 mg once daily and then increase by 30 mg after 1 week as tolerated up to 120 mg daily
Venlafaxine	Inhibition of serotonin and norepinephrine reuptake	Nausea, hypertension at high dosages	Cardiac disease, hypertension, use of tramadol	Improvement of depression and generalized anxiety, improvement of sleep	A. Diabetic neuropathy	37.5 mg once or twice daily/225 mg daily	Increase by 37.5–75 mg each week as tolerated

(*continued*)

Table 9.1.1 Continued

Drug	Main Mechanisms of Action	Common Major Side Effects	Precautions	Other Benefits	Efficacy: Level A/B Rating[a]	Starting Dose/ Maximum Dose	Titration
Calcium channel $\alpha_2\delta$ ligands							
Gabapentin	Acts on $\alpha_2\delta$ subunit of voltage-gated calcium channels, which decreases central sensitization	Sedation, dizziness, peripheral edema, weight gain	Reduce dosages in renal insufficiency	No clinically significant drug interactions, improvement of generalized anxiety and sleep	A. Diabetic neuropathy, PHN, cancer neuropathic pain B. Spinal cord injury pain	100–300 mg once to 3 times daily/1200 mg 3 times daily	Increase by 100–300 mg 3 times daily every 3 to 7 days as tolerated
Pregabalin	Acts on $\alpha_2\delta$ subunit of voltage-gated calcium channels, which decreases central sensitization	Sedation, dizziness, peripheral edema, weight gain	Reduce dosages in renal insufficiency	No clinically significant drug interactions, improvement of generalized anxiety and sleep	A. Diabetic neuropathy, PHN, spinal cord injury	25–75 mg once daily/300 mg twice daily	Increase by 75 mg daily after 3–7 days and then by 150 mg every 3–7 days as tolerated
Topical lidocaine							
Lidocaine 5% plasters	Block of sodium channels	Local erythema, itch, rash	None	No systemic side effects, potential effect on allodynia	A. PHN	1–3 patches/3 patches	None

Capsaicine patches 8%	TRPV1 agonist	Pain Erythema Elevated blood pressure due to initial increase in pain	None	No systemic side effects—potential effects on burning pain, itch, and allodynia	A. HIV neuropathy and PHN	1–4 patches to cover the painful area—repeat every 3 months	None
Opioid agonists							
Tramadol	Mu receptor agonist and inhibition of monoamine reuptake	Nausea and vomiting, constipation, dizziness, somnolence	History of substance abuse, suicide risk, use of antidepressants in elderly patients	Rapid onset of analgesic effect, effect on inflammatory pain	A. Diabetic neuropathy, phantom pain B. Spinal cord injury	50 mg once or twice daily/400 mg daily as long-acting drug	Increase by 50–100 mg every 3–7 days
Morphine Oxycodone Methadone Levorphanol	Mu receptor agonists (oxycodone may also cause κ-receptor antagonism)	Nausea and vomiting, constipation, dizziness, somnolence	History of substance abuse, suicide risk, risk of misuse on long-term use	Rapid onset of analgesic effect, effect on inflammatory pain	A. Diabetic neuropathy, PHN, phantom pain	10–15 mg morphine every 4 h or as needed (equianalgesic doses for other opioids)/ up to 300 mg morphine has been used in neuropathic pain	After 1–2 weeks convert to long-acting opioids, use short-acting drugs as needed and as tolerated

Abbreviations: ECG, electrocardiogram; HIV, human immunodeficiency virus; PHN, postherpetic neuralgia; TRPV1, transient receptor potential vanilloid receptor-1.
[a]Recommendation grading: Level A = good scientific evidence from several Class I trials; Level B = some scientific evidence from Class II trials (lower-class trials).
[a]Data modified from references [7, 9, 12].

1 week. In general, high doses of venlafaxine (150–225 mg/day) are effective to alleviate NP.

$\alpha_2\delta$ ligand agonists

The efficacy of gabapentin and pregabalin is established in diabetic PPN and PHN [14, 15]. The analgesic effect is mainly related to a decrease in central sensitization and nociceptive transmission through action on the $\alpha_2\delta$ subunit of calcium channels [7, 8]. Effective dosages for NP are 1800–3600 mg/day for gabapentin and 150–600 mg/day for pregabalin (with inconsistent effects of 150 mg/day). Extended-release formulations of gabapentin (gabapentin ER or gabapentin enacarbil) are also effective [6]. In clinical studies, pregabalin has usually been initiated at 150 mg/day, but initial doses of 75 mg/day at bedtime are recommended to reduce side effects, especially for older patients or those with significant comorbidities or polypharmacy. Both drugs need individual titration, with a shorter titration schedule for pregabalin (upward increase by 75 mg every 3 days). Individual titration should be performed up to efficacy and side effects. Gabapentin is generally administered three times per day (except for gabapentin extended release), whereas pregabalin should be administered twice per day. More information on various anticonvulsants used as adjuvant analgesics is provided in Chapter 4.

Lidocaine 5% medicated plasters

The efficacy of lidocaine 5% plasters is established mainly in PHN. Lidocaine plasters may reduce ectopic discharges through its sodium channel-blocking properties. However, on the basis of a meta-analysis, the therapeutic gain is very modest compared with placebo [17], and one recent trial using an enriched enrollment design failed to show a difference between lidocaine and placebo on the primary outcome measure [18]. Lidocaine 5% medicated plasters are generally safe and have little systemic absorption; only local adverse effects (eg, mild skin reactions) have been reported [18]. Up to four plasters per day for a maximum of 12 hours within a 24-hour period is usually recommended to cover the painful area, but longer applications for up to 24 hours have been found to be safe. Titration is not necessary.

Tramadol

The efficacy of tramadol, including the combination with acetaminophen, is established predominantly in diabetic PPN [7, 8, 10–12]. Tramadol may induce dizziness, dry mouth, nausea, constipation, and somnolence and can cause or aggravate cognitive impairment, particularly in the elderly. Although the risk of abuse is lower than with other opioids, tramadol should be used with caution in patients with a history of substance abuse. There is an increased risk of seizures in patients with epilepsy or those receiving drugs that reduce the seizure threshold, such as TCAs. Serotonin syndrome may occur if tramadol is used in combination with other serotonergic medications (particularly selective serotonin reuptake inhibitors, but also other antidepressants) (see Chapter 10). Tramadol should be initiated at low dosages, particularly in elderly patients (50 mg once daily), and then titrated as tolerated. Effective dosages range from 200 to 400 mg/day. Dose reduction is recommended in older patients and those with renal impairment or cirrhosis.

Opioids

The use of opioids for the treatment of chronic pain has increased dramatically over the past decade. There has been a longstanding debate about their efficacy in chronic NP [19]. However, several randomized controlled trials (RCTs) have now established that opioids (oxycodone, methadone, morphine) have efficacy in diabetic PPN and PHN at dosages ranging from 10 to 120 mg for oxycodone, the most studied drug in NP [7–9, 11, 12]. The dosages necessary to reach efficacy may be higher for NP than for nociceptive pain. Furthermore, the effects obtained with NP are not necessarily associated with significant improvement in quality of life, psychological comorbidities, and sleep disorders. Another opioid, tapentadol (500 mg daily), a μ-opioid agonist with norepinephrine reuptake inhibition, has been more recently studied in peripheral NP with encouraging effects in one diabetic NP trial.

The most common side effects of opioids are constipation, sedation, nausea, dizziness, and vomiting, although these generally decrease after long-term treatment, with the exception of constipation [20]. Opioids must be used with great caution in patients with a history of drug abuse.

The problems associated with long-term opioid use are increasingly reported in chronic noncancer pain. Long-term morphine administration may be associated with immunologic changes and hypogonadism [10]. The risk of misuse or addiction in chronic pain, although low (2.6%) in recent systematic studies [21], may represent a concern in long-term use. Prescription opioid dependence is associated with structural and functional changes in brain regions implicated in the regulation of affect, reward, and motivational functions [22]. Opioid-induced hyperalgesia, defined as an increase in pain sensitivity with the use of opioids, has been demonstrated in animal models, and there is concern that it might occur in humans [23]. For these reasons, opioids are considered to be second-line treatment for noncancer NP, including NP, in all current recommendations [7, 10, 24].

Capsaicin patches

Capsaicin is an agonist of transient receptor potential vanilloid receptor-1 (TRPV1) and activates TRPV1 ligand-gated channels on nociceptive fibers. This activity in turn causes depolarization, the initiation of an action potential, and the transmission of pain signals to the spinal cord [25]. After several days of application, TRPV1-containing sensory axons are desensitized, a process also referred to as "defunctionalization." Standard capsaicin-containing creams (0.075%) have been found to be moderately effective for PHN, but they require many applications per day and cause a burning sensation for many days before the analgesic effect starts.

The efficacy of a single application of high-concentration capsaicin patch (8%) for 30 minutes compared with a low concentration patch (0.04%) has been demonstrated from weeks 2 to 12 in PHN or human immunodeficiency virus (HIV) neuropathy [5, 26, 27] with confirmed safety in an open-label 48-week extension [26, 28, 29]. However, the optimal duration of the patches to produce analgesic efficacy was distinct in PHN (60 minutes) and HIV neuropathy (30 minutes). The effects of this treatment on multiple symptoms that may be particularly sensitive to this drug, including mechanical allodynia, itch or burning pain, were not addressed.

Adverse effects were primarily due to capsaicin-related reactions at the application site (pain, erythema, sometimes edema, and itching). Initial pain often necessitated opioids, and blood pressure should be carefully monitored because of the potential risk of high blood pressure during application (probably due to severe pain in some patients). The drug does not produce impairment of standard sensory evaluation in PHN and HIV neuropathy after repeated applications for up to one year [29]. In a subset of patients in the controlled trial of painful HIV neuropathy [29], the high-concentration capsaicin patch produced no change in sequential quantitative sensory testing (QST) measures, including thresholds for vibration, heat pain, and cooling. In human volunteers, only a transient (1 week) impairment of epidermal nerve fiber density was noted by skin punch biopsy after a single application, but there was a 93% recovery after 6 months [28]. However, it is not clear whether these data are applicable to patients with peripheral nerve lesions after repeated applications. In PHN, the high-concentration capsaicin patch may be applied for 30 minutes (feet) to 60 minutes (other areas) to the painful area, up to a maximum of 4 patches, and should not be applied to the face.

Capsaicin patches have not been considered so far in evidence-based therapeutic recommendations but should probably be proposed for patients with focal neuropathy particularly when there are concerns with systemic side effects, compliance with the treatment, or drug-drug interactions. Patients with burning pain, itch, and allodynia to mechanical or heat stimuli might be the best candidates for such treatment.

Other drug treatments

Antiepileptics other than gabapentin and prégabaline have been infrequently studied in NP, with the notable exception of carbamazepine in trigeminal neuralgia. Trials of other anticonvulsants (eg, topiramate, oxcarbazepine, carbamazepine, lacosamide) have generally demonstrated mild or discrepant effects in large-scale RCTs. Initial data about valproate are still controversial [7, 11], despite positive RCTs in diabetic NP and PHN [7, 11, 24].

In summary, TCAs, pregabalin/gabapentin, and duloxetine are generally indicated as first-line treatment for NP [7, 10] (Figure 9.1.1). However, in diabetic neuropathy, recommendations for first-line treatment diverge: the American Academy of Neurology recommends pregabalin as first-line treatment [24], and the United Kingdom National Institute for Clinical Excellence recommends duloxetine [31]. Lidocaine plasters, with their excellent tolerability, are recommended as first-line treatment for PHN. Second-line therapy includes strong opioids or tramadol, and third-line treatments include other antiepileptics [7, 10].

Other neuropathic pain indications

Several trials have been recently performed in central NP, particularly SCI pain. These trials have confirmed the benefit of pregabalin for SCI pain [7, 32] but not for poststroke pain [33], whereas lower-class trials suggested the benefit of TCAs, gabapentin, and tramadol for SCI pain.

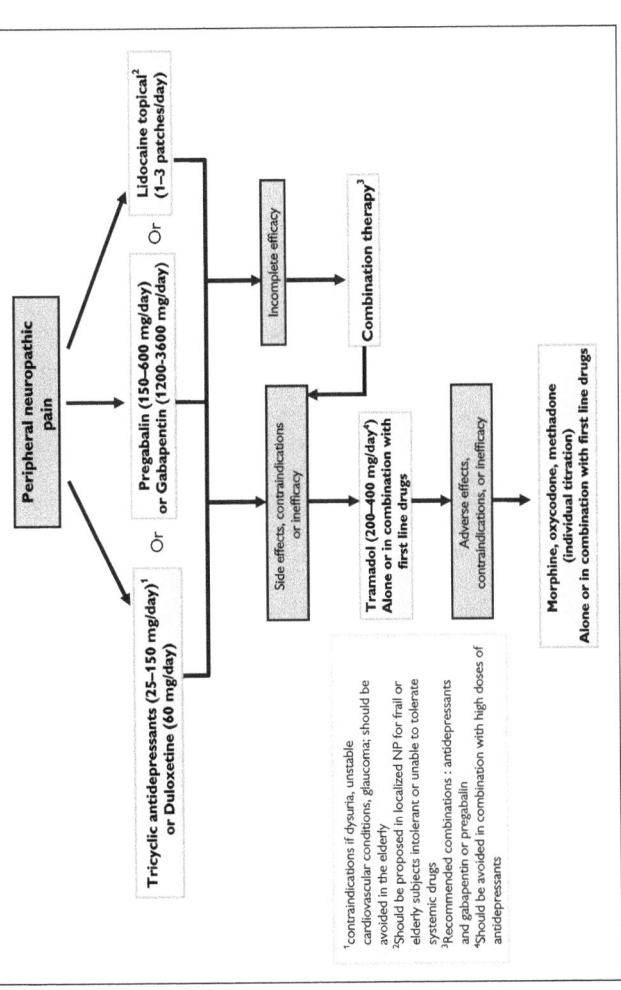

Figure 9.1.1 Therapeutic algorithm proposed for peripheral neuropathic pain (NP) in clinical practice. This algorithm is based on current evidence-based recommendations and systematic reviews in peripheral NP [7, 9, 11, 30]. Serotonin–norepinephrine reuptake inhibitor (SNRI) antidepressants are generally recommended as first choice, but duloxetine has higher evidence for peripheral NP. The choice between first-line drugs depends on the clinical profile (for example, tricyclic antidepressants should be avoided in the elderly), contraindications, and comorbid conditions (for example, patients with anxiety, sleep disorders, or depression may benefit more from pregabalin/gabapentin or SNRI antidepressants). Capsaicin high-concentration patches have not been considered yet in this therapeutic algorithm.

Pregabalin is now the drug of choice for SCI pain. One comparative trial found efficacy of high-dose levorphanol for central pain [7]. A Class I trial showed no superiority of duloxetine over placebo on the primary outcome of central pain due to stroke or SCI, but several secondary outcomes, including allodynia to brush and cold, favored duloxetine [34]. Thus, central NP seems to generally respond to the same drug treatments as peripheral NP.

Several large-scale trials of posttraumatic neuropathy have been reported. One trial found that gabapentin (up to 2400 mg/day) had no effect on pain intensity but improved pain relief, sleep, and quality of life [35]. Another trial found that pregabalin was moderately effective (difference 0.62 versus placebo) on the primary outcome [36]. Lower-class studies found moderate effects of amitriptyline and low-dose venlafaxine on postmastectomy pain and discrepant results with topical capsaicin [7].

Studies of gabapentin have found positive results in GuillainBarré syndrome and cancer NP and discrepant results in phantom limb pain. Opioids and tramadol have been found to be efficacious for phantom limb pain, and amitriptyline has been found to be efficacious for cancer NP [7, 10, 11].

Human immunodeficiency virus neuropathy and chronic radiculopathy have generally been found to be poorly responsive to drugs that are useful for other NP conditions. In HIV neuropathy, negative results were obtained with amitriptyline, topical lidocaine, gabapentin [7, 9, 11], and pregabalin [37], whereas lamotrigine, smoked cannabis, and more recently high-concentration capsaicin patches (see below) were found to be moderately useful.

A recent large-scale study using an enrichment phase demonstrated no benefit of pregabalin for lumbosacral radiculopathy [7]. A crossover placebo-controlled study of nortriptyline, morphine, and their combination in lumbosacral radiculopathy was negative for the primary outcome and found only slight effects for the combination of worst pain and pain relief [38]. However, given the lack of specific assessment of pain quality in most trials, the possibility that these drugs might be effective in a subset of patients exhibiting particular clinical phenotypes or improve only some dimensions of NP cannot be excluded. New studies are warranted for these indications, particularly among patients with failed back syndrome, because a large subset of these patients have NP, and radicular pain probably represents one of the most common NP conditions in the general population [2].

Combination and head-to-head studies

Several head-to-head comparative studies have been performed in NP, but most studies are single-center trials with small sample size. Most initial studies aimed to compare drugs from the same class, particularly TCAs. These trials found similar efficacy of different TCAs [7, 10, 11]. In one study, venlafaxine 225 mg/day was equivalent to imipramine 150 mg/day with respect to overall pain intensity and tolerability, but it was less effective on the proportion of responders, pain relief, and quality of life [7]. Other trials reported similar efficacy of gabapentin and nortriptyline in diabetic NP and PHN [39], pregabalin and amitriptyline [40] and lamotrigine and amitriptyline in diabetic NP [41]. These results may be related to small sample size and do not exclude the possibility that these drugs have distinct effects depending on patients' clinical profiles, which were generally not detailed at baseline.

Several placebo-controlled trials confirmed the benefit of gabapentin combined with nortriptyline or morphine compared with gabapentin monotherapy in a mixed group of patients with diabetic PPN and PHN [39, 42, 43]. The combination drug arms demonstrated better efficacy with lower dosages compared with monotherapy without an increase in side effects. Similarly, in diabetic NP, gabapentin in combination with oxycodone was superior to gabapentin alone [43]. In a large-scale study, patients unresponsive to moderate dosages of pregabalin (300 mg daily) or duloxetine (60 mg daily) were subsequently randomized to receive either the combination of both drugs at similar dosages or increased dosages of the same drugs in monotherapy (ie, 600 mg of pregabalin or 120 mg of duloxetine) [44]. The study showed similar efficacy of combination therapy and monotherapy at high dosages on primary and secondary outcomes, including quality of life and sleep and no significant difference in side effects. These trials suggest that combination therapy with these agents may be useful, particularly when monotherapy is incompletely effective.

Newer drug treatments for neuropathic pain

More recently, three drug classes have been studied in RCTs involving NP.

Botulinum toxin type A

Several lines of investigation have suggested that botulinum toxin type A (BTX-A), a potent neurotoxin commonly used for the treatment of focal muscle hyperactivity, may have analgesic effects independent of its action on muscle tone, possibly by acting on neurogenic inflammation [45]. Such mechanisms may be involved in some cases of peripheral NP. Several single-center RCTs reported the long-term efficacy of a series of subcutaneous injections of BTX-A (from 100 to 200 units) injected into the painful area among patients with mononeuropathies (traumatic or related to herpes zoster [46]) and patients with diabetic PPN [47], but one unpublished study in post-herpetic neuralgia was negative [48]. It is interesting to note that in two studies, the onset of efficacy (approximately 1 week) and duration of effects (3 months) was remarkably similar. The drug had an excellent safety profile; patients reported only pain during injection and no systemic side effects. One study found that a possible predictor for response to BTX-A was the preservation of warm thresholds [44]. These data indicate a need for large-scale trials with this compound in peripheral NP. Novel preparations of BTX-A with selective activity on afferent sensory fibers are under development.

Cannabinoids

The therapeutic potential of cannabinoids has been extensively investigated in chronic pain after the discovery of cannabinoid receptors and their endogenous ligands. Oromucosal cannabinoids (2.7 mg Δ-9-tetrahydrocannabinol/2.5 mg cannabidiol) have been found to be effective in multiple sclerosis-associated pain and for refractory peripheral

NP associated with allodynia [7, 10, 11], but several unpublished trials are negative. Adverse events include dizziness, dry mouth, sedation, fatigue, gastrointestinal effects, and oral discomfort. Although no impairment of cognition or psychoactive effects were noted in these trials, cannabis may exacerbate psychiatric conditions, so cannabinoids are not recommended for patients with psychiatric disorders. There is controversy with regard to tolerance and dependence after long-term treatment [49]. Oromucosal cannabinoids are currently not available for the treatment of NP in the United States, but they are available in Canada.

Improving therapeutic outcome in neuropathic pain

Despite newer drugs and the increased use of rational polypharmacy that may improve therapeutic response, the response to most treatments for NP is generally modest. The number needed to treat for 50% pain relief (the number of patients necessary to treat to obtain one responder compared with placebo) ranges from 3 to 6 in recent clinical trials of pregabalin, gabapentin, SNRIs, and opioids for peripheral NP [11]. One contributor to these findings is the large placebo effects in recent trials [50]. Another reason may be related to the fact that psychological comorbid conditions are generally insufficiently taken into account in RCTs. For example, it has been found that catastrophizing plays a role in the persistence of pain in PHN [51] and in the predicted pain-related disability (independent of pain severity) in NP [52]. It is possible that maladaptive coping and catastrophizing tend to be associated with a poor response to drugs. The most important issue probably relates to the methodology of the trials. In particular, RCTs performed in NP may have failed to identify responder profiles to therapy mostly because they did not take into account the heterogeneity of NP syndromes, which include a variety of symptoms (ie, burning pain, electric shocks, brush-evoked pain) and symptom combinations that are presumably linked to distinct mechanisms [8, 53, 54]. The assessment of symptoms and signs in clinical trials is best performed with specific assessment questionnaires and an extension of the clinical examination, such as QST [6]. For example, some studies have reported in post hoc analyses that patients with mechanical (static or dynamic) allodynia were better responders to systemic sodium channel blockers or pregabalin [53]. These studies suggest the importance of differentiating patients with and without evoked pain for therapeutic studies.

In addition, preservation of thermal sensation has been associated with a better outcome with topical therapy. Classification of patients with sensory profiles based on specific NP questionnaires and QST rather than etiology could reduce pathophysiologic heterogeneity within study groups and increase the positive treatment responses [8, 53, 6].

Conclusions

Consensus recommendations for the pharmacologic treatment of NP generally suggest antiepileptics (notably pregabalin) and TCAs (notably amitriptyline) as first-line therapy; SNRIs (duloxetine) and lidocaine 5% plasters are also proposed as first-line agents in certain NP conditions. Clinical advances in the management of NP include the implementation of comparative studies and combination therapy trials, the study of rarer and often neglected NP conditions, and the identification of responder profiles based on a detailed characterization of symptoms and signs using sensory examination and specific pain questionnaires. New drug treatments will undoubtedly contribute to the improved management of NP.

References

1. Treede RD, Jensen TS, Campbell JN, et al. Neuropathic pain: redefinition and a grading system for clinical and research purposes. Neurology 2008; 70:1630–1635.

2. Bouhassira D, Lantéeri-Minet M, Attal N, et al. Prevalence of chronic pain with neuropathic characteristics in the general population. Pain 2008; 136:380–387.

3. Bouhassira D, Attal N. Diagnosis and assessment of neuropathic pain: the saga of clinical tools. Pain 2011; 152(3 Suppl):S74–S83.

4. Attal N, Fermanian C, Fermanian J, et al. Neuropathic pain: are there distinct subtypes depending on the aetiology or anatomical lesion? Pain 2008; 138:343–353.

5. Backonja M, Wallace MS, Blonsky ER, et al. NGX-4010 C116 Study Group. NGX-4010, a high concentration capsaicin patch, for the treatment of postherpetic neuralgia: a randomised, double-blind study. Lancet Neurol 2008; 7:1106–1112.

6. Haanpää M, Attal N, Backonja M, et al. NeuPsig NeuPSIG guidelines on neuropathic pain assessment. Pain 2011; 152:14–27.

7. Attal N, Cruccu G, Baron R, et al; European Federation of Neurological Societies. EFNS guidelines on the pharmacological treatment of neuropathic pain. 2010 revision. Eur J Neurol 2010; 17:1113-e88.

8. Baron R, Binder A, Wasner G. Neuropathic pain: diagnosis, pathophysiological mechanisms, and treatment. Lancet Neurol 2010; 9:807–819.

9. Dworkin RH, O'Connor AB, Backonja M, et al. Pharmacologic management of neuropathic pain: evidence evidence-based recommendations. Pain 2007; 132:237–251.

10. Dworkin RH, O'Connor AB, Audette J, et al. Recommendations for the pharmacological management of neuropathic pain: an overview and literature update. Mayo Clin Proc 2010; 85(3 Suppl):S3–S14.

11. Finnerup NB, Sindrup SH, Jensen TS. The evidence for pharmacological treatment of neuropathic pain. Pain 2010; 150:573–581.

12. Baron R, Freynhagen R, Töolle T, et al. The efficacy and safety of pregabalin in the treatment of neuropathic pain associated with lumbosacral radiculopathy. Pain 2010; 150:420–427.

13. Gahimer J, Wernicke J, Yalcin I, et al. A retrospective pooled analysis of duloxetine safety in 23,983 subjects. Curr Med Res Opin 2007; 23:175–184.

14. Freeman R, Durso-Decruz E, Emir B. Efficacy, safety and tolerability of pregabalin treatment for painful diabetic peripheral neuropathy: findings from seven randomized controlled trials accross a range of doses. Diabetes Care 2008; 31:1448–1454.

15. Wiffen PJ, McQuay HJ, Edwards JE, et al. Gabapentin for acute and chronic pain. Cochrane Database Syst Rev 2009. Available at http://onlinelibrary.wiley.com/doi/10.1002/14651858.CD005452.pub2/pdf. Accessed 27 November, 2014.

16. Irving G, Jensen M, Cramer M, et al. Efficacy and tolerability of gastric-retentive gabapentin for the treatment of postherpetic neuralgia: results of a double-blind, randomized, placebo-controlled clinical trial. Clin J Pain 2009; 25:185–192.

17. Khaliq W, Alam S, Puri N. Topical lidocaine for the treatment of postherpetic neuralgia. Cochrane Database Syst Rev 2007; 18:CD004846.

18. Baron R, Mayoral V, Leijon G, et al. 5% lidocaine medicated plaster versus pregabalin in post-herpetic neuralgia and diabetic polyneuropathy: an open-label, non-inferiority two-stage RCT study. Curr Med Res Opin 2009; 25:1663–1676.

19. Eisenberg E, McNicol ED, Carr DB. Efficacy and safety of opioid agonists in the treatment of neuropathic pain of nonmalignant origin: systematic review and meta-analysis of randomized controlled trials. JAMA 2005; 293:3043–3052.

20. Moore RA, McQuay HJ. Prevalence of opioid adverse events in chronic non-malignant pain: systematic review of randomised trials of oral opioids. Arthritis Res Ther 2005; 7:R1046–R1051.

21. Portenoy RK, Farrar JT, Backonja MM, et al. Long-term use of controlled-release oxycodone for noncancer pain: results of a 3-year registry study. Clin J Pain 2007; 23:287–299.

22. Upadhyay J, Maleki N, Potter J, et al. Alterations in brain structure and functional connectivity in prescription opioid-dependent patients. Brain 2010; 133(pt 7):2098–2114.

23. Crofford LJ. Adverse effects of chronic opioid therapy for chronic musculoskeletal pain. Nat Rev Rheumatol 2010; 6:191–197.

24. Bril V, England J, Franklin GM, et al. Evidence-based guideline: treatment of painful diabetic neuropathy: report of the American Academy of Neurology, the American Association of Neuromuscular and Electrodiagnostic Medicine, and the American Academy of Physical Medicine and Rehabilitation. Neurology 2011; 76:1758–1765.

25. Wong GY, Gavva NR. Therapeutic potential of vanilloid receptor TRPV1 agonists and antagonists as analgesics: Recent advances and setbacks. Brain Res Rev 2009; 60:267–277.

26. Backonja MM, Malan TP, Vanhove GF, et al. NGX-4010, a high-concentration capsaicin patch, for the treatment of postherpetic neuralgia: a randomized, double-blind, controlled study with an open-label extension. Pain Med 2010; 11:600–608.

27. Simpson DM, Brown S, Tobias J. Controlled trial of high-concentration capsaicin patch for treatment of painful HIV neuropathy. Neurology 2008; 70:2305–2313.

28. Kennedy WR, Vanhove GF, Lu SP, et al. A randomized, controlled, open-label study of the long-term effects of NGX-4010, a high-concentration capsaicin

28. ...patch, on epidermal nerve fiber density and sensory function in healthy volunteers. J Pain 2010; 11:579–587.
29. Simpson DM, Gazda S, Brown S, et al. Long-term safety of NGX-4010, a high-concentration capsaicin patch, in patients with peripheral neuropathic pain. J Pain Symptom Manage 2010; 39:1053–1064.
30. Attal N, Cruccu G, Haanpää M, et al. EFNS guidelines on pharmacological treatment of neuropathic pain. Eur J Neurol 2006; 13:1153–1169.
31. Tan T, Barry P, Reken S. Pharmacological management of neuropathic pain in non-specialist settings: summary of NICE guidance. Br Med J 2010; 340:c1079.
32. Vranken JH, Dijkgraaf MG, Kruis MR, et al. Pregabalin in patients with central neuropathic pain: a randomized, double-blind, placebo-controlled trial of a flexible-dose regimen. Pain 2008; 136:150–157.
33. Kim JS, Bashford G, Murphy TK, et al. Safety and efficacy of pregabalin in patients with central post-stroke pain. Pain 2011; 152:1018–1023.
34. Vranken J, Hollmann MW, van der Vegt MH, et al. Duloxetine in patients with central neuropathic pain: a a randomized, double-blind, placebo-controlled trial of a flexible-dose regimen. Pain 2010; 152:267–273.
35. Gordh TE, Stubhaug A, Jensen TS, et al. Gabapentin in traumatic nerve injury pain: a randomized, double-blind, placebo-controlled, cross-over, multi-center study. Pain 2008; 138:255–266.
36. van Seventer R, Bach FW, Toth CC, et al. Pregabalin in the treatment of post-traumatic peripheral neuropathic pain: a randomized double-blind trial. Eur J Neurol 2010; 17:1082–1089.
37. Simpson DM, Schifitto G, Clifford DB. Pregabalin for painful HIV neuropathy: a randomized, double-blind, placebo-controlled trial. Neurology 2010; 74:413–20.
38. Khoromi S, Cui L, Nackers L, et al. Morphine, nortriptyline and their combination vs. placebo in patients with chronic lumbar root pain. Pain 2007; 130:66–75.
39. Gilron I, Baley JM, Tu D, et al. Nortritpyline and gabapentin, alone and in combination for neuropathic pain: a double-blind, randomised controlled crossover trial. Lancet 2009; 374:1252–1261.
40. Bansal D, Bhansali A, Hota D, et al. Amitriptyline versus vs. pregabalin in painful diabetic neuropathy: a randomized double blind clinical trial. Diabet Med 2009; 26:1019–1026.
41. Jose VM, Bhansali A, Hota D, et al. Randomized double-blind study comparing the efficacy and safety of lamotrigine and amitriptyline in painful diabetic neuropathy. Diabet Med 2007; 24:377–383.
42. Gilron I, Bailey JM, Tu D, et al. Morphine, gabapentin, or their combination for neuropathic pain. N Engl J Med 2005; 352:1324–1334.
43. Hanna M, O'Brien C, Wilson MC. Prolonged-release oxycodone enhances the effects of existing gabapentin therapy in painful diabetic neuropathy patients. Eur J Pain 2008; 12:804–813.
44. Tesfaye S, Wilhelm S, Lledo A, et al. Duloxetine and pregabalin: high-dose monotherapy or their combination? The "COMBO-DN study"—a multinational, randomized, double-blind, parallel-group study in patients with diabetic peripheral neuropathic pain. Pain 2013; 154:2616–2625.
45. Ranoux D, Attal N, Morain F, et al. Botulinum toxin type a A induces direct analgesic effects in chronic neuropathic pain: a double blind placebo controlled study. Ann Neurol 2008; 64:274–283.

46. Xiao L, Mackey S, Hui H, et al. Subcutaneous injection of botulinum toxin a is beneficial in postherpetic neuralgia. Pain Med 2010; 11:1827–1833.

47. Yuan RY, Sheu JJ, Yu JM, et al. Botulinum toxin for diabetic neuropathic pain: a randomized double-blind crossover trial. Neurol 2009; 72:1473–1478.

48. 19 1622-066: A Multicenter, Double-Blind, Randomized, Placebo-Controlled, Parallel Study of the Safety and Efficacy of BOTOX (Botulinum Toxin Type A) Purified Neurotoxin Complex in Subjects with Postherpetic Neuralgia (PHN). Available at: http://www.allerganclinicaltrials.com/pdfs/neuroscience/Results_Web_Posting191622-066.pdf. Accessed 22 May 2014.

49. Manzanares J, Julian M, Carrascosa A. Role of the cannabinoid system in pain control and therapeutic implications for the management of acute and chronic pain episodes. Curr Neuropharmacol 2006; 4:239–257.

50. Katz J, Finnerup NB, Dworkin RH. Clinical trial outcome in neuropathic pain: relationship to study characteristics. Neurology 2008; 70:263–272.

51. Haythornthwaite JA, Clark MR, Pappagallo M, et al. Pain coping strategies play a role in the persistence of pain in post-herpetic neuralgia. Pain 2003; 106:453–460.

52. Sullivan MJ, Lynch ME, Clark AJ. Dimensions of catastrophic thinking associated with pain experience and disability in patients with neuropathic pain conditions. Pain 2005; 113:310–315.

53. Attal N, Bouhassira D, Baron R, et al. Assessing symptom profiles in neuropathic pain clinical trials: Can can it improve outcome? Eur J Pain 2011; 15:441–443.

54. Bouhassira D, Attal N. Novel strategies for neuropathic pain. In: Villanueva L, Dickenson A, Ollat H, eds. *The Pain System in Normal and Pathological States: A Primer for Clinicians. Progress in Pain Research and Management.* Vol. 1. Seattle, WA: IASP Press; 2004.

Chapter 9.2

Cancer-related Pain

Paul N. Luong and Russell K. Portenoy

Introduction

Pain is highly prevalent in the cancer population, occurring in approximately one-third of those receiving active therapy and approximately two-thirds of those with advanced illness [1]. Cancer-related pain also occurs in the large and heterogeneous group of survivors, but its epidemiology is yet poorly defined in this population. Although numerous barriers may contribute to undertreatment [2], several evidence-based guidelines have been developed to provide guidance on appropriate cancer-related pain management. Opioid-based therapy is widely accepted as the first-line strategy for moderate or severe chronic pain due to active cancer, and it is usually considered to be a second-line approach for those with limited or absent disease. Nonopioid analgesics are first-line treatments for some types of pains, and when opioids are provided, they may be combined with these agents to yield additive effects and reduce the impact of undertreatment.

In the treatment of pain related to active cancer, adjuvant analgesics usually are added to opioid therapy after the opioid dose has been titrated to optimize the balance between analgesic and adverse effects. The occurrence of troublesome adverse effects before satisfactory analgesia occurs characterizes the pain as "poorly responsive" to the specific opioid and route of administration, and a trial of one or more adjuvant analgesics is a common strategy to address this scenario [3].

The decision to offer a trial of an adjuvant analgesic to address poor opioid responsiveness must be based on the findings of a comprehensive assessment of the pain and the patient [4]. Rational decisions require an understanding of the nature of the pain, status of the underlying disease, and its treatment, salient medical and psychiatric comorbidities, psychosocial factors, and the values and preferences of the patient and family.

Types of adjuvant analgesics

There have been few studies of the adjuvant analgesics in populations with cancer pain, and their use has been based largely on data obtained from studies in other populations and clinical experience [5]. Some drug classes seem to have potential utility in heterogeneous painful conditions and have been described as "multipurpose" adjuvant analgesics. Others have been used specifically for specific conditions, such as neuropathic pain, bone pain, musculoskeletal pain, or pain and other symptoms in bowel obstruction [Table 9.2.1] [5].

Table 9.2.1 Adjuvant Analgesics Used for Cancer Pain (adapted from Lussier, Huskey, and Portenoy [6])

Category Based on Conventional Use	Class	Subclass	Drugs
Multipurpose analgesics	Antidepressants	Tricyclics	amitriptyline, desipramine, nortriptyline
		SNRIs	duloxetine, minalcipran, venlafaxine, desvenlafaxine
		SSRIs	paroxetine, citalopram
		Other	buproprion
	Corticosteroids	–	dexamethasone, prednisone, methylprednisone
	α_2-Adrenergic agonists	–	tizanidine, clonidine
	Cannabinoids	–	dronabinol, nabilone, nabiximols
	Topical analgesics	–	local anesthetics, capsaicin, tricyclic antidepressants, NSAIDs, others
Used for neuropathic pain	All multipurpose analgesics	See above	see above
	Anticonvulsants	–	gabapentin, pregabalin, divalproex, phenytoin, carbamazepine, oxcarbazepine, topiramate, lamotrigine,
	Sodium channel blockers	Sodium channel modulator	lacosamide
		Sodium channel blocker	mexiletine, IV lidocaine
	N-Methyl-D-aspartate receptor antagonists	–	ketamine, memantine, dextromethorphan, amantadine

(continued)

Table 9.2.1 Continued

Category Based on Conventional Use	Class	Subclass	Drugs
	GABA agonists	GABA$_a$ agonists	clonazepam
		GABA$_b$ agonists	baclofen
Used for bone pain	Osteoclast inhibitors	Bisphosphonates	pamidronate, zolendronate, ibandronate
		–	calcitonin
	Radiopharmaceuticals	–	strontium-89, samarium-153
	Plus: NSAIDs, corticosteroids		
Used for bowel obstruction	Anticholinergic drugs	–	scopolamine, atropine, glycopyrrolate
	Somatostatin analogue	–	octreotide
	Plus: Corticosteroids		

Abbreviations: IV, intravenous; NSAIDs, nonsteroidal anti-inflammatory drugs; SNRI, serotonin-norepinephrine reuptake inhibitor; SSRI, selective serotonin reuptake inhibitor.

Multipurpose analgesics

The so-called multipurpose analgesics include antidepressants, corticosteroids, α_2-adrenergic agonists, cannabinoids, and topical therapies. As noted, the population of cancer survivors is best considered to be comparable with other populations with chronic pain. For these patients, some of the multipurpose adjuvant analgesics, such as the antidepressants and topical therapies, are considered first-line approaches. For those with active cancer, all of these drugs are typically considered as add-on therapies for any type of pain that is poorly opioid-responsive. In practice, the usual indication is neuropathic pain that has been poorly responsive to an opioid.

Analgesic antidepressants

Among many available antidepressants, analgesic efficacy is best established for some of the tricyclic compounds and the serotonin-norepinephrine reuptake inhibitors (SNRIs) [Table 9.2.1]. Evidence of analgesic efficacy in cancer-related pain is very limited, however. The tricyclic antidepressants have been suggested to have some analgesic efficacy in a few partially controlled trials [7, 8] and one randomized controlled trial of amitriptyline [9]. Although the side effects associated with the tricyclic drugs may be of concern in medically ill patients, some patients may have symptoms other than pain that may benefit from specific side effects, such as sedation. The secondary amine tricyclic drugs, such as desipramine, have fewer side effects than the tertiary amine drugs such as amitriptyline, and former agents are usually preferred when pain is the target symptom.

Serotonin-norepinephrine reuptake inhibitors are usually better tolerated than tricyclics and have been shown to be analgesic in a few cancer-related conditions. Venlafaxine can decrease acute neurosensory symptoms and chronic oxaliplatin neurotoxicity when administered during 2-week course of chemotherapy [10]. It can also prevent chronic postmastectomy pain when initiated the night before surgery and administered for two weeks [11]. Duloxetine was effective in relieving pain from chronic oxaliplatin-induced peripheral neuropathy in 63% of patients with colon cancer who could tolerate it [12], as well as in patients who did not tolerate pregabalin [13]. Relief of chemotherapy-induced peripheral neuropathy was also shown in a recent randomized controlled trial [14].

There is no evidence of analgesic efficacy of all other antidepressants in cancer-related pain. Bupropion, which is associated with less fatigue and somnolence than either the tricyclic drugs or the SNRIs, might nevertheless be a good option for cancer patients who also are experiencing distressing sedation or fatigue. Mirtazapine, which has no evidence of pain relief, has been shown to improve sleep, anxiety, and depression in cancer patients, and it can be used to address these symptoms [15].

When used to treat cancer-related pain, antidepressants should be prescribed using the same doses and protocols applied in the treatment of chronic noncancer pain syndromes. These are described in Chapter 3.

Corticosteroids

Corticosteroids have been widely used to treat cancer-related symptoms such as pain, nausea, fatigue, poor appetite, malaise, and poor overall quality of life [15]. Although evidence from clinical trials is limited, there is extensive clinical experience that suggests benefit for varied pain syndromes related to active cancer, including neuropathic pain resulting from nerve compression, bone pain, pain associated with capsular expansion or duct obstruction, pain from bowel obstruction, pain caused by lymphedema, and headache caused by increased intracranial pressure [16]. The mechanism of action is unknown, but it may relate to the reduction of peritumoral edema, anti-inflammatory effects, and direct effects on nociceptive neural systems.

Although many clinicians favor dexamethasone, presumably because of its relatively low mineralocorticoid effects, there are no comparative trials of the various drugs in this class. Prednisone and methylprednisolone are acceptable alternatives.

In the setting of advanced cancer, a corticosteroid typically is added to opioid therapy at a low dose, with no intent to taper or discontinue therapy. The risks of long-term treatment, which includes myopathy, immunosuppression, psychotomimetic effects, and hypoadrenalism, are less relevant when life expectancy is short. When life expectancy is indeterminate or relatively long, these potential adverse effects must be considered; open-ended treatment with a corticosteroid should not be undertaken unless safer alternatives are lacking.

There are no data that adequately inform dose selection for long-term corticosteroid therapy in those with advanced cancer. Typically, dexamethasone 1–2 mg/day or prednisone 5–10 mg/day is administered [Table 9.2.2]. Dexamethasone can be given orally or parenterally, and the low-dose regimen may be initiated with a larger loading dose of 10–20 mg.

Based on experience in the treatment of emergent spinal cord compression [17], a high-dose dexamethasone regimen has been used to treat very severe and escalating pain (sometimes called "pain emergencies"). A dexamethasone loading dose of 50–100 mg intravenously may be followed by 12–24 mg four times daily, which is tapered over 1–3 weeks, usually as some other intervention (eg, radiotherapy or a pain intervention such as neural blockade) is used to treat the pain.

α_2-Adrenergic agonists

Clonidine and tizanidine are α_2-adrenergic agonists. Clonidine has been used in diverse types of chronic pain; intraspinal clonidine has been shown to reduce neuropathic pain in patients with severe cancer pain partly responding

Table 9.2.2 Therapeutic Dose Ranges for Commonly Used Adjuvant Analgesics (adapted from Lussier, Huskey, and Portenoy [6])

Category Based on Conventional Use	Class	Drugs	Usual Starting Dose	Usual Effective Dose Range
Multipurpose analgesics	Antidepressants	Doses similar to use for chronic noncancer pain (Chapter 3)		
	Corticosteroids	dexamethasone	1–2 mg qd-bid or larger loading dose of 10–20 mg	1–2 mg qd-bid, PO or IV. Higher dose can be used for pain emergencies (see text)
		prednisone		5–10 mg qd-bid
	α_2-Adrenergic agonists	tizanidine	1–2 mg qhs	2–8 mg bid
Used for neuropathic pain	see Chapter 9.1			
Used for bone pain	Osteoclast inhibitors	pamidronate	–	60–90 mg qmonth
		calcitonin	–	1 unit/kg per day
Used for bowel obstruction	Anticholinergic drugs	glycopyrrolate	0.1 mg qd	0.1–0.2 mg tid
	Somatostatin analog	octreotide	Varies	0.1–0.3 mg bid

Abbreviations: bid, twice a day; IV, intravenously; PO, orally; q, each; qd, once a day; qhs, every night at bedtime; tid, three times a day.

to opioids [18]. Tizanidine, which is approved for the treatment of spasticity, has demonstrated analgesic efficacy in myofascial pain syndrome and chronic headache. Presumably, these analgesic effects, like those of clonidine, relate to increased activity in monoamine-dependent, endogenous pain modulating pathways in the spinal cord and brain.

The use of α_2 agonists as adjuvant analgesics is limited by their side effects, which include dry mouth, somnolence, and orthostatic hypotension. A trial of one of these drugs is usually considered only after other adjuvant analgesics have proved ineffective. Tizanidine has less hypotensive effects and may be preferred over clonidine for a trial in cancer patients with opioid-refractory neuropathic pain. It may be initiated at 1–2 mg at night, and the dose is then gradually escalated while monitoring analgesia and adverse effects.

Cannabinoids

An oromucosal spray containing tetrahydrocannabinol (THC) plus cannabidiol (and smaller concentrations of other compounds), known as nabiximols, is undergoing worldwide development and has already been approved in several countries for opioid-refractory pain due to cancer [19]. A trial of a commercially available drug (eg, dronabinol [THC] or nabilone) is typically considered only in those patients who are refractory to opioids and other appropriate adjuvant analgesics. The advent of nabiximols may alter the positioning of these compounds relative to other adjuvants. All cannabinoids should be started at a relatively low initial dose at night and titrated up if tolerated.

Topical analgesics

Creams and patches containing local anesthetics, capsaicin preparations, nonsteroidal anti-inflammatory drugs, tricyclic compounds, or other drugs are available commercially or may be compounded, singly or in combination. Low-dose topical capsaicin (0.1%) was shown to relieve pain from painful mononeuropathies and polyneuropathies, including peripheral painful mononeuropathies after cancer surgery (postmastectomy, postthoracotomy, postamputation) [20]. Other topical analgesics have not been tested specifically for cancer-related pain, but the favorable risk profiles of these formulations justifies the effort to identify a useful formulation when pain has a limited distribution. Sequential trials should be considered, based on the approach used to manage chronic noncancer pain (see Chapter 8).

Adjuvant analgesics used for neuropathic pain

Adjuvant analgesics are commonly used to treat cancer-related neuropathic pain. As discussed above, they are empirically used as add-on therapy in populations with active disease when pain is poorly responsive to the opioid regimen, and they are commonly considered first-line for neuropathic pain in cancer survivors. In the latter context, these patients are treated like those populations with chronic neuropathic pain unrelated to cancer (see Chapter 9.1).

First-line therapies for neuropathic pain include two of the multipurpose analgesics—the analgesic antidepressants and the topical agents—and the gabapentinoids (see below). The antidepressants typically are considered first if comorbid depression exists.

Anticonvulsant analgesics

The analgesic effects of the gabapentinoids are well established. In cancer-related neuropathic pain, evidence is best for pregabalin. This drug relieved neuropathic cancer pain in a randomized controlled trial, and it was better than gabapentin or amitriptyline [9]. It also reduced the symptoms of chemotherapy-induced peripheral neuropathy [21]. Studies of gabapentin have demonstrated its analgesic efficacy in chemotherapy-induced peripheral neuropathy and diverse types of neuropathic cancer pain [9]. Combination of gabapentin and an opioid was shown to be more effective than the opioid alone [22, 23].It also worked in combination with imipramine (low-dose gabapentin 200 mg bid and imipramine 10 mg bid were more effective and better tolerated than high-dose gabapentin 400 mg bid alone) [24]. When combined with topical EMLA cream, gabapentin also decreased acute pain and prevented chronic pain after mastectomy [25].

Patients may respond to either pregabalin, gabapentin, or both drugs. Given the lack of evidence for analgesic efficacy of other anticonvulsants in neuropathic cancer pain, trials of other drugs should be considered after a patient demonstrates lack of benefit from both of the gabapentinoids and one or more analgesic antidepressant drugs. In this setting of refractory neuropathic pain, other anticonvulsants (and other drug classes described below) may be considered. These include oxcarbazepine, lamotrigine, lacosamide, topiramate, and sodium divalproex.

Other drugs used for neuropathic pain

In addition to the other drugs categorized as multipurpose analgesics—such as tizanidine or a cannabinoid—several drug classes also are considered for refractory cancer-related neuropathic pain. These include sodium channel blockers and N-methyl-D-aspartate (NMDA) receptor antagonists.

Sodium channel blockade has been recognized as an analgesic mechanism for decades. A brief intravenous infusion of lidocaine has been shown to be effective to relieve diverse types of noncancer neuropathic pain, but all trials in cancer pain have failed to show analgesic efficacy. Nevertheless, it can be considered in severe refractory neuropathic cancer pain, either as a brief intravenous infusion or long-term continuous subcutaneous administration [26].

The NMDA receptor is involved in both the sensitization of central neurons and the functioning of the opioid receptor. Although a large randomized controlled trial [27] did not confirm the efficacy of ketamine, a recent review concluded on the basis of five randomized controlled trials that this drug should be considered for patients with cancer pain that has not responded adequately to standard therapy [28]. The drug is usually administered as a continuous intravenous or subcutaneous infusion. A broad range of doses has been used, beginning as low as 0.05 mg/kg per hour; most clinicians seem to favor a starting dose of 0.2–0.5 mg/kg per hour. The infusion is gradually increased, often until benefit occurs or side effects appear. Concurrent treatment with a benzodiazepine or neuroleptic is usually done to reduce the risk of psychotomimetic effects. Oral ketamine has also been used, and based on clinical experience, a starting dose of 0.5 mg/kg in two or three divided doses is used. This is titrated higher, again seeking an analgesic effect with tolerable side effects. A benzodiazepine or neuroleptic drug is coadministered.

Other NMDA receptor antagonists, such as memantine, amantadine, and dextromethorphan, have also been studied in diverse types of neuropathic pain, but results have been mixed. They are rarely considered for trials in cancer-related neuropathic pain that has not responded to other therapies.

Other drugs that are sometimes used for noncancer pain syndromes with a neuropathic component can be considered for treatment-refractory cancer-related neuropathic pain. The $GABA_A$ agonist, clonazepam, and the $GABA_B$ agonist, baclofen, are two such agents.

Drugs used for bone pain

The assessment of a patient with bone pain may suggest the need for radiation therapy or an intervention such as kyphoplasty or surgery. Patients with multifocal pain are usually managed with a nonsteroidal anti-inflammatory drug, opioid, and adjuvant analgesics used specifically for bone pain. In addition to a corticosteroid, such as dexamethasone, drugs to consider in this setting include bisphosphonates, calcitonin, and bone-seeking radionuclides [Table 9.2.1]. New human monoclonal antibodies (mAbs) that inhibit the so-called receptor activator of nuclear factor κB ligand (RANKL) are also approved in the United States for the treatment of skeletal-related events, of which bone pain is one.

Osteoclast inhibitors

Bisphosphonates have been shown to be useful in preventing skeletal-related events, including fracture and pain, and may improve the quality of life in cancer patients with bone metastases [29]. They act by directly inhibiting osteoclast activity, stimulating osteoblasts to produce osteoclast-inhibiting factor, and causing osteoclast apoptosis. Substantial research supports the analgesic potential of all of the parenteral drugs, including pamidronate, zolendronate, ibandronate, and clodronate, and oral ibandronate and clodronate [29]. Comparative data are very limited, and the selection of a specific drug is usually based on experience, cost, and convenience.

Bisphosphonate administration may be accompanied by flu-like symptoms, a transient decline in renal function, and symptomatic hypocalcemia. A laboratory screening is important before treatment to exclude or limit dosing in those with renal insufficiency or low-serum calcium levels. Repeated administration of a bisphosphonate has been associated with more serious complications, specifically osteonecrosis of the jaw [30] and atypical femoral fractures. Given the evidence that oral trauma and dental infections increase the risk of osteonecrosis, an alternative strategy for bone pain should be considered for patients with very poor dentition, jaw infection, or recent substantial dental procedures.

There is conflicting information about the potential for subcutaneous calcitonin to reduce metastatic bone pain [31]. Given the limited evidence, an empirical trial of this treatment is generally considered only when other treatments are not available or are ineffective.

Radionuclides

Bone-seeking radionuclides, such as strontium-89 and samarium-153, link a short-lived radiation source to a bisphosphonate molecule. The drug is taken up at the site of bone metastases and can be a useful treatment for refractory multifocal bone pain [3]. Bone marrow suppression is a significant concern, however, and treatment requires specialized skills and facilities.

Human monoclonal antibodies

In a recent comparative, randomized, double-blinded study, denosumab, a human mAb against RANKL, was shown to be better than zoledronic acid for prevention of skeletal-related complications, including pathologic fractures and spinal cord compression, in men with bone metastases from prostate cancer [32]. This and other mAb compounds are being studied for their analgesic profiles and may contribute to the management of bone pain in the future.

Drugs used for the pain of bowel obstruction

When malignant bowel obstruction is not surgically remediable, the need to control pain and other obstructive symptoms (eg, distention, nausea, and vomiting) becomes very important. Management usually considers removal of gastric contents (via oral or nasogastric suction, or venting gastrostomy), hydration, and pain control using opioids and adjuvant analgesics. Adjuvant analgesics may have direct effects on pain or reduce pain and other symptoms by lessening peritumoral edema (corticosteroids) or diminishing intraluminal secretions and peristaltic movements (anticholinergic drugs and octreotide).

Anticholinergic drugs

Anticholinergic drugs reduce propulsive and nonpropulsive gut motility and decrease intraluminal secretions. Scopolamine can be administered by a transdermal patch, a convenient route for those with limited gastrointestinal absorption [33, 34]. In many countries, scopolamine is available only as the hydrobromide salt, which crosses the blood-brain barrier and may produce central nervous system side effects, such as somnolence and confusion. Glycopyrrolate has a pharmacological profile similar to scopolamine but has minimal penetration through the blood-brain barrier. Although never systematically evaluated as a treatment for the symptoms of bowel obstruction, a trial of glycopyrrolate may be warranted in those who are predisposed to these side effects.

Octreotide

Octreotide is a somatostatin analog that inhibits gastric, pancreatic, and intestinal secretions and reduces motility. This drug may also relieve pain and other symptoms in bowel obstruction [33, 34]. Octreotide has a good safety profile and may be administered as repeated subcutaneous boluses or as a continuous infusion. A long-acting subcutaneous formulation is also available. Dosing usually starts at 100 mcg subcutaneously twice daily, but it can be titrated to much higher levels. Cost may be prohibitive, however.

Conclusions

Adjuvant analgesics are important additions to opioid therapy in pain related to active cancer and often are first-line strategies for cancer-related pain in the survivor community. The development of these drugs during recent decades has been very rapid, and there now are numerous drugs in many classes. The clinical approach to the selection and administration of one or more of these drugs in populations with cancer remains largely empirical, based on data obtained in other populations and experience. Studies that compare the safety and effectiveness of these drugs in various indications are badly needed.

References

1. van den Beuken-van Everdingen MH, de Rijke JM, Kessels AG, et al. Prevalence of pain in patients with caner: a systematic review of the past 40 years. Ann Oncol 2007; 18:1437–1449.
2. Deandrea S, Montanari M, Moja L, Apolone G. Prevalence of undertreatment in cancer pain. A review of published literature. Ann Oncol 2008; 19:1985–1991.
3. Mercadante S, Portenoy RK. Opioid poorly responsive cancer pain. Part 3: Clinical strategies to improve opioid responsiveness. J Pain Symptom Manage 2001; 21:338–354.
4. Dworkin RH, O'Connor AB, Backonja M, et al. Pharmacologic management of neuropathic pain: evidence-based recommendations. Pain 2007; 132:237–251.
5. Lussier D, Portenoy RK. Adjuvant analgesics in pain management. In: Hanks G, Cherny NI, Christakis N, et al, eds. *Oxford Textbook of Palliative Medicine*. 4th ed. Oxford, England: Oxford University Press; 2010: pp. 706–734.
6. Lussier D, Huskey AG, Portenoy RK. Adjuvant analgesics in cancer pain management. Oncologist 2004; 9:571–591.
7. Ventafridda V, Bonezzi C, Caraceni A, et al. Antidepressants for cancer pain and other painful syndromes with deafferentation component: comparison of amitriptyline and trazodone. Ital J Neurol Sci 1987; 8:579–587.
8. Walsh TD. Controlled study of imipramine and morphine in chronic pain due to advanced cancer. Proc Am Soc Clin Oncol 1986; 5:237.
9. Mishra S, Bhatnagar S, Goyal GN, et al. A comparative efficacy of amitriptyline, gabapentin, and pregabalin in neuropathic cancer pain: a prospective randomized double-blind placebo-controlled study. Am J Hosp Pall Care 2012; 29:177–182.
10. Durand JP, Deplanque G, Montheil V, et al. Efficacy of venlafaxine for the prevention and relief of oxaliplatin-induced acute neurotoxicity: results of

EFFOX, a randomized, double-blind, placebo-controlled phase III trial. Ann Oncol 2012; 23:200–205.

11. Reuben SS, Makari-Judson G, Lurie SD. Evaluation of efficacy of the perioperative administration of venlafaxine XL for the prevention of postmastectomy pain syndrome. J Pain Symptom Manage 2004; 27:133–139.

12. Yang YH, Lin JK, Chen WS, et al. Duloxetine improves oxaliplatin-induced neuropathy in patients with colorectal cancer: an open-label pilot study. Supp Care Cancer 2012; 20:1491–1497.

13. Matsuoka H, Makimura C, Koyama A, et al. Pilot study of duloxetine for cancer patients with neuropathic pain non-responsive to pregabalin. Anticancer Res 2012; 32:1805–1809.

14. Smith EM, Pang H, Cirrincione C, et al. Effect of duloxetine on pain, function, and quality of life among patients with chemotherapy-induced painful peripheral neuropathy: a randomized clinical trial. JAMA 2013; 309:1359–1367.

15. Cankurtaran ES, Ozalp E, Soygur H, et al. Mirtazapine improves sleep and lowers anxiety and depression in cancer patients: superiority over imipramine. Supp Care Cancer 2008; 16:1291–1298.

16. Mercadante SL, Berchovich M, Casuccio A, et al. A prospective randomized study of corticosteroids as adjuvant drugs to opioids in advanced cancer patients. Am J Hosp Palliat Care 2007; 24:13–19.

17. Loblaw DA, Perry J, Chambers A. Systematic review of the diagnosis and management of malignant extradural spinal cord compression: the Cancer Care Ontario Practice Guidelines Initiative's Neuro-Oncology Disease Site Group. J Clin Oncol 2005; 23:2028–2037.

18. Eisenach JC, DuPen S, Dubois M, et al. Epidural clonidine analgesia for intractable cancer pain: the Epidural Clonidine Study Group. Pain 1995; 61:391–399.

19. Russo EB, Guy GW, Robson PJ. Cannabis, pain, and sleep: lessons from therapeutic clinical trials of Sativex, a cannabis-based medicine. Chem Biodivers 2007; 4:1729–1743.

20. Ellison N, Loprinzi CL, Kugler J, et al. Phase III placebo-controlled trial of capsaicin cream in the management of surgical neuropathic pain in cancer patients. J Clin Oncol 1997; 15:2974–2980.

21. Saif MW, Syrigos K, Kaley K, Isufi I. Role of pregabalin in treatment of oxaliplatin-induced sensory neuropathy. Anticancer Res 2010; 30:2927–2933.

22. Caraceni A, Zecca E, Bonezzi C, et al. Gabapentin for neuropathic cancer pain: a randomized controlled trial from the Gabapentin Cancer Pain Study Group. J Clin Oncol 2004; 22:2909–2917.

23. Keskinbora K, Pekel AF, Aydinli I. Gabapentin and an opioid combination versus opioid alone for the management of neuropathic cancer pain: a randomized open trial. J Pain Symptom Manage 2007; 34:183–189.

24. Arai YC, Matsubara T, Shimo K, et al. Low-dose gabapentin as useful adjuvant to opioids for neuropathic cancer pain when combined with low-dose imipramine. J Anesthesiol 2010; 24:407–410.

25. Fassoulaki A, Triga A, Melemeni A, Sarantopoulos C. Multimodal analgesia with gabapentin and local anesthetics prevents acute and chronic pain after breast surgery for cancer. Anesth Analg 2005; 101:1427–1432.

26. Brose WG, Cousins MJ. Subcutaneous lidocaine for treatment of neuropathic cancer pain. Pain 1991; 45:145–148.

27. Hardy J, Quinn S, Fazekas B, et al. Randomized, double-blind, placebo-controlled study to assess the efficacy and toxicity of subcutaneous ketamine in the management of cancer pain. J Clin Oncol 2012; 30:3611–3617.

28. Bredlau AL, Thakur R, Korones DN, Dworkin RH. Ketamine for pain in adults and children with cancer: a systematic review and synthesis of the literature. Pain Med 2013; 14:1505–1517.

29. Body JJ. Bisphosphonates for malignancy-related bone disease: current status, future developments. Support Care Cancer 2006; 14:408–418.

30. Woo SB, Hellstein JW, Kalmar JR. Systematic review: bisphosphonates and osteonecrosis of the jaw. Ann Intern Med 2006; 144:753–761.

31. Martinez-Zapata MJ, Roque M, Alonso-Coello P. Calcitonin for metastatic bone pain. Cochrane Rev 2006; (3):CD003223.

32. Fizazi K, Carducci M, Smith M, et al. Denosumab versus zoledronic acid for treatment of bone metastases in men with castration-resistant prostate cancer: a randomized, double-blind study. Lancet 2011; 377:813–822.

33. Ripamonti C, Mercadante S, Groff L, et al. Role of octreotide, scopolamine butylbromide, and hydration in symptom control of patients with inoperable bowel obstruction and nasogastric tubes: a prospective randomized trial. J Pain Symptom Manage 2000; 19:23–34.

34. Mercadante S, Ripamonti C, Casuccio A, et al. Comparison of octreotide and hyoscine butylbromide in controlling gastrointestinal symptoms due to malignant inoperable bowel obstruction. Supp Care Cancer 2000; 8:188–191.

Chapter 9.3

Rheumatic Pain and Fibromyalgia

Mary-Ann Fitzcharles

Introduction

The understanding of pain processes in rheumatic conditions has changed considerably over the past decade. There is emerging evidence that neurological mechanisms contribute to the pain experience in rheumatic pain, originally believed to be driven by nociceptive mechanisms only [1, 2]. This new knowledge is partly due to the recognition that fibromyalgia (FM) is a pain syndrome with pathogenesis centered in the nervous system, rather than a condition of soft tissue abnormality, and that there is considerable overlap between FM and defined rheumatic conditions.

When the pain due to osteoarthritis (OA) and inflammatory arthritis (IA) was believed to be purely nociceptive, treatments directed towards the peripheral process that included nonsteroidal anti-inflammatory drugs (NSAIDs) and opioids were appropriate choices. With this new appreciation of pain mechanisms, treatment options directed to pain management will be more diverse. Therefore, a logical step is to explore use of adjuvant medications, previously used only for neuropathic pain, in rheumatic pain management. With promising effect in FM, adjuvant agents may eventually be useful in management of a wider spectrum of rheumatic pain conditions. Adjuvant agents with US Food and Drug Administration (FDA) approval for treatment of FM are pregabalin, duloxetine, and milnacipran, with duloxetine also approved for treatment of low back and OA pain [3, 4].

Rheumatic conditions causing pain

Rheumatic pain may arise in the soft tissues, the joints, or muscles and bones. Soft-tissue rheumatism comprises conditions affecting tendons, their insertions, and bursae and is the most prevalent reason for musculoskeletal pain. Pain arising in these tissues will be experienced by almost all individuals at some time in life. Conditions affecting joints may be divided into those categorized as OA, with pathology originating in the cartilage, or IA with inflammatory changes predominantly in the synovial tissue and secondary changes in cartilage and bone. Fibromyalgia in contrast is a neurologically based condition, without peripheral tissue abnormality that may be present as a unique entity or associated with some other rheumatic disease. Increasing numbers of patients with arthritis are now recognized to be manifesting symptoms of sensitization of pain pathways both in the periphery and centrally.

Neurogenic mechanisms in rheumatic conditions

Pain due to a rheumatic process is a complex interaction of local factors at the periphery, modulation of the pain message by plastic changes in the spinal cord and brain stem, altered function in the brain, and finally effects mediated via the descending inhibitory system [5]. Local tissue changes cause activation of the primary somatosensory neuron and account for the initial nociceptive response. In the setting of ongoing pain, this initial response is followed by neurophysiologic and even structural changes within the nervous system.

Several lines of evidence strengthen the hypothesis of interplay of neurogenic factors in the pain experience of rheumatic conditions. In the setting of continued pain, neuronal peripheral and central sensitization leads to an exaggeration of response to various stimuli, and is a factor in perpetuation of pain [5]. Molecules augmenting the pain message include glutamate, substance P, and calcitonin gene-related peptide, whereas those that mostly dampen the pain message are the endogenous opioids, cannabinoids, serotonin, and norepinephrine [5–7]. Changes in brain function and structure have been observed in patients with painful OA, with (1) reversal of activation after administration of lidocaine into the painful joint and (2) return of thalamus to normal size after joint replacement [8–11].

Adjuvant treatments

In the light of the contribution of neurogenic mechanisms in rheumatic pain, as well as the considerable overlap with FM in many rheumatic conditions, the effect of adjuvant treatments is of interest. Two broad categories of adjuvant medications, namely anticonvulsants and antidepressants, have been extensively studied in FM. Anticonvulsant agents dampen neuronal hyperexcitability with effect on sensitization, whereas the antidepressant group affects descending pain inhibitory pathways in the brain stem and spinal cord via serotonin and norepinephrine mechanisms [12, 13]. Adjuvants may also have the added advantage of affecting some of the common accompaniments to pain such as anxiety, depression, and sleep disturbance. Table 9.3.1 provides a summary of the evidence of analgesic efficacy for various adjuvant analgesics for the treatment of FM and rheumatic pain along with recommended doses.

Analgesic anticonvulsant drugs

Anticonvulsant drugs in the class of gabapentinoids ($\alpha_2\delta$ ligand drugs) are classified as second-generation anticonvulsants, and they have shown clinical efficacy in the treatment of FM [14, 15]. In a meta-analysis of treatment effects of gabapentin and pregabalin in FM, there was strong evidence for reduction

Table 9.3.1 Adjuvant Pharmacotherapy for Fibromyalgia and Rheumatic Pain

Drug Class		Fibromyalgia	Suggested Daily Dose	Rheumatic Pain	Suggested Daily Dose
Anticonvulsants	Gabapentin	+	100–300 mg HS	No studies	N/A
	Pregabalin	+	25–100 mg HS	No studies	N/A
Antidepressants	TCAs	+	10–25 mg HS	No studies	N/A
	SSRIs	+/–	Variable	No studies	N/A
	SNRIs				
	duloxetine	+	30–60 mg	+	30–60 mg
	milnacipran	+	100–200 mg	–	N/A
Topical agents	NSAIDs	No studies	N/A	+	TID/QID
	Capsaicin	No studies	N/A	+	TID
Cannabinoids	Herbal	No studies	N/A	No studies	N/A
	Nabilone	+	0.5–1 mg	No studies	N/A
	Sativex	No studies	N/A	+	2–8 puffs

Abbreviations: HS, at bedtime; N/A, data not available; NSAIDs, nonsteroidal anti-inflammatory drugs; SNRIs, serotonin norepinephrine reuptake inhibitors; SSRIs, selective serotonin reuptake inhibitors; TCAs, tricyclic antidepressants; TID, 3 times a day; QID, 4 times a day; +, evidence supports analgesic efficacy; –, evidence suggests does not have analgesic efficacy; +/–, conflicting evidence on analgesic efficacy.

of pain, improved sleep, and improved health-related quality of life, and some impact on fatigue and anxiety [14]. Troublesome side effects of drowsiness, weight gain, and edema have led physicians to reduce doses in clinical practice, in contrast to the higher doses used in clinical trials [3, 4].

To date, there have been no controlled studies examining the use of gabapentinoids in human rheumatic diseases, although pain behaviors were reduced by pregabalin administration in an OA rat model [16]. Only one small post hoc clinical study has reported beneficial effects of pregabalin in OA of the hip [17]. Extrapolating from experience in FM, but without study in arthritic disease, these agents are used off-label to treat both pain and sleep disturbance in arthritis patients. Combination drug treatment is also commonly used in clinical practice and may allow for lower doses of individual drugs, thereby attenuating side effects. A single study has reported better effect when a combination of pregabalin and celecoxib, a cyclooxygenase-2 inhibitor, was used compared with monotherapy for the treatment of back pain [18].

Pain modulators affecting descending inhibitory pathways

Although mostly recognized for effect on descending pain inhibitory pathways in the brain stem and spinal cord, mediated by norepinephrine and serotonin, antidepressants may also have an impact on opioid mechanisms, ion channels, N-methyl-D-aspartate (NMDA) channels, and even inflammation. In a mouse model of rheumatoid arthritis (RA), both citalopram and fluoxetine inhibited disease progression and also inhibited production of inflammatory cytokines in human synovial membrane cultures [19].

Although clinical studies are mostly in FM, there is evidence for effect in other rheumatic conditions in which analgesics and NSAIDs are not sufficiently effective [20]. The best studied in this group are the older tricyclic antidepressants (TCAs). Amitriptyline and its metabolite nortriptyline have shown efficacy in the treatment of FM but with modest effect that tends to wear off over time [21]. However, the selective serotonin reuptake inhibitors (SSRIs) have not shown consistent analgesic effect [22]. In a meta-analysis of nine trials, antidepressants in the TCA and SSRI classes improved pain but not function in patients with chronic low back pain [23].

The development of new antidepressant agents with reduced side-effect profile holds promise for the management of rheumatic pain. Newer antidepressants that inhibit reuptake of serotonin and norepinephrine, termed serotonin norepinephrine reuptake inhibitors, may offer improved tolerability and have shown promise in pain management. Duloxetine and milnacipran, agents with a balanced effect on serotonin and norepinephrine, have shown consistent improvement in pain and function in FM, with sustained response up to one year [24–30]. Both duloxetine and milnacipran have been approved by the FDA for treatment of FM, and duloxetine has an added indication for the treatment of chronic pain including low back pain. However, dosing for duloxetine is lower than that for depression, with effect mostly seen with a daily dose of 60 mg/day. Although the primary outcome for most of these studies has focused on pain relief, improvements in global health status, mood, and even fatigue have been reported. The ideal dosing of these agents will likely be clarified as physicians become more comfortable with use but will probably be somewhat flexible [31].

The use of antidepressant medications for pain modulation in rheumatology clinical practice, other than FM, is still preliminary. The most common reason for caution is the concern for drug interactions, problems of tolerability in patients with other comorbidities, and especially the effect of these agents in older patients.

The cannabinoids

Contrary to popular belief, the cannabinoid effects are not only confined to the nervous system and pain pathways, but they have an impact on inflammation and even joint damage [32]. Information regarding the use of cannabinoids for management of pain in musculoskeletal conditions is available from preclinical science, population surveys, anecdotal reports, and the results of only three formal clinical trials: two in FM and one in RA [33–38].

Treatment of musculoskeletal pain is a common reason for use of medicinal cannabis, with 80% of users in a pain clinic in the United States reporting myofascial pain, and up to one third of persons in two population studies in the United Kingdom and Australia reporting use for treatment of arthritis pain [33, 34, 39]. A concerning issue raised by both the population studies is the overlap of recreational and medicinal cannabinoid use. Healthcare professionals need to clarify to patients that any recommendation for herbal cannabis use can only be made specifically for the purpose of symptom management. In addition, it is necessary that persons using medicinal cannabis must discriminate between recreational and medicinal use. The fine line that exists between use and abuse has medicolegal implications for any healthcare professional caring for patients who use medicinal cannabis.

The effect of nabilone, a synthetic cannabinoid, has been studied in two small randomized controlled trials in patients with FM [37, 38]. In the first study, nabilone was associated with improved pain and function, whereas the second study reported equivalency of nabilone and amitriptyline for effect on sleep but without significant effect on either pain or quality of life. Both studies reported more side effects in those using nabilone. In an uncontrolled study, pain scores were reduced two hours after herbal cannabis use in 28 FM patients but with no impact upon function as measured by the Short Form 36 Health Survey or the FIQ [40]. Therefore, on the strength of evidence, cannabinoid use in FM remains of questionable value.

Cannabinoids have been studied in RA in a single randomized controlled trial [36]. Fifty-eight RA patients were treated with the oromucosal spray Sativex or placebo over a 5-week period, with significant improvement in pain and sleep in the active group. This first study of cannabinoid treatment in an inflammatory rheumatic disease suggests a possible therapeutic role, but additional study is required.

In a systematic review and meta-analysis that included 4 studies with 218 patients with musculoskeletal disease, pain scores showed statistical improvements, but side effects of drowsiness and confusion were common with numbers needed to harm reported as four and nine, respectively [41]. With considerable limitations of studies with small sample sizes, short study duration, and effect sizes noted to be modest at best, any conclusions remain tenuous and require further study.

Topical and intra-articular treatments

Although topical agents have been used to treat rheumatic pain for decades, the resurgence of interest in the recent past deserves comment. Topical treatments may be simple counterirritants such as menthol, NSAIDs, anesthetic agents such as ketamine, topical TCAs, and capsaicin, each with different mechanisms of action [42–46]: capsaicin depletes substance P from nerve endings after repeated application for approximately 3 weeks, counterirritants make use of gate mechanisms of pain modulation, and NSAIDs inhibit peripheral inflammatory mediators. Prolonged cutaneous analgesia has been demonstrated in the rat model by the application of amitriptyline, an agent that affects sodium channels and therefore the pain response [47].

These agents provide an attractive alternative to oral treatments with increasing evidence for effects on peripheral mechanisms of nociception and with the added advantage of reduced systemic effects [48]. Local and systemic absorption can vary depending upon the formulation used, but generally plasma levels of drug are low, whereas local tissue concentrations can be high [49, 50]. Therefore the side-effect profile of a topical agent is more favorable than for an orally administered treatment. Topical NSAIDs have a better effect than placebo in management of a single joint OA or acute muscle injuries but no effect in chronic low back pain or FM [51]. It also seems that the analgesic effect of topical NSAIDs is apparent within the first two weeks of treatment, with less obvious effect thereafter [52].

For the last half-century, injection of corticosteroids into bursae, tendon sheaths, and joints has been a useful and enduring treatment strategy for rheumatic conditions. The advantage of local injections is that the dose of corticosteroid is modest and almost without systemic effect, success rate is acceptable, and importantly, the risks are minimal [53, 54]. The two greatest concerns are for (1) introduction of infection into a tissue space and (2) rupture of a tendon when inadvertently the tendon rather than the tendon sheath is injected, both of which are mostly rare occurrences.

In studies of joint injections of corticosteroids, the effect is mostly of short duration, with no evidence for long-term effect on pain or natural history of disease [55]. In contrast, injections of corticosteroids into soft tissues structures are more efficacious in initiating prolonged improvement of symptoms [56]. Repeated treatments may be required after several months, with anecdotal recommendations to limit the number of injections to three for each location over a one-year period.

Intra-articular or intralesional injections may be considered as locally applied treatments [55]. Corticosteroid are the most commonly used agent, but with some interest in the use of botulinum toxin, or simply a local anesthetic agent. Intra-articular hyaluronic acid may have a role in the treatment of knee OA in selected patients [57, 58]. Even though hyaluronic acid is cleared from the joint within 24 hours, the postulated mechanism of action is a change in chondrocyte cell function and cartilage metabolism. This treatment has been shown to be effective, safe, and well tolerated, with most favorable effects within the first three months of treatment [59].

Herbal and Diet

Herbal treatments and dietary manipulations are commonly used by patients with rheumatic disease, mostly not prescribed by physicians and often without evidence for efficacy [60, 61]. A recent review from Japan reported that of the 260 complementary products available for arthritis treatment in Japan, only 41 had been tested in controlled trials [62]. In a systematic review of the use of herbal medicine for the treatment of OA, several agents including phytodolor, capsaisin, evening primrose oil, devil's claw (harpargophytum), and avocado/soya have been reported to have some effect on pain in patients with OA [63, 64]. Although studies have not reported severe side effects, and herbal agents seem to be relatively safe, caution needs to be exercised regarding interaction with other prescribed medications.

Dietary supplementation with omega 3 polyunsaturated fatty acids (eg, alpha linolenic acid) has been shown to possess anti-inflammatory properties and has been associated with reduction in consumption of NSAIDs in RA [65]. Both glucosamine and chondroitin sulphate are used extensively by patients with OA, although a recent meta-analysis indicates no reduction in pain or joint space narrowing when compared with placebo [66]. The healthcare professional should acknowledge that disclosure by the patient of use of complementary products speaks to a trusting doctor-patient relationship and may even view the exploration of other treatment options as a positive effort on the part of the patient to improve health.

Other agents

There are a number of agents, each with unique mechanisms of action, which may have some use in pain management, although evidence in rheumatic diseases other than FM hardly exists. The categories of drugs included are the dopaminergic agents, NMDA receptor antagonists, and 5-hydroxytryptamine-3 receptor antagonists. Anti-Parkinsonian drugs that augment dopamine are an effective treatment for restless legs, a frequent accompaniment to rheumatic pain conditions. A small study that examined the effect of pramipexole in FM reported improvement in symptoms of pain, although use is tempered by frequent gastrointestinal side effects [67].

Because activation of the NMDA receptor is a mechanism by which chronic pain is perpetuated, blockade of this receptor would be highly desirable in patients with chronic pain. However, there are no studies examining this treatment strategy in musculoskeletal pain [68].

The 5-hydroxytryptamine-3 receptor antagonists are agents that have been primarily used as antiemetic drugs. In a recent study of patients with FM, dolasetron infused monthly over a period of three months resulted in significant reduction in pain intensity compared with placebo and showed a good safety profile [69]. Once again, there are no studies in other rheumatic pain conditions, and effects in FM must still be considered to be preliminary.

Summary

The notion to consider adjuvant agent use in rheumatic conditions stems from the knowledge of neurogenic mechanisms in FM and the overlap of FM type pain in rheumatic disease. These agents, apart from topical applications, have mostly not been adequately studied in rheumatic conditions, but they have been tentatively used in clinical practice. In line with the diverse effects of some of the adjuvant agents, with impact on sleep, mood, and even fatigue, they may eventually be used more commonly in rheumatic diseases and not only for treatment of FM. Benefits related to use of oral agents, especially for the older population, need to be carefully weighed against potential risks before adjuvants can be universally recommended for routine pain management.

References

1. Clauw DJ, Witter J. Pain and rheumatology: thinking outside the joint. Arthritis Rheum 2009; 60:321–324.
2. Fitzcharles MA, Almahrezi A, Shir Y. Pain: understanding and challenges for the rheumatologist. Arthritis Rheum 2005; 52:3685–3692.
3. Goldenberg DL, Clauw DJ, Fitzcharles MA. New concepts in pain research and pain management of the rheumatic diseases. Semin Arthritis Rheum 2011; 41:319–34.
4. Boomershine CS, Crofford LJ. A symptom-based approach to pharmacologic management of fibromyalgia. Nat Rev Rheumatol 2009; 5:191–199.
5. McDougall JJ. Arthritis and pain. Neurogenic origin of joint pain. Arthritis Res Ther 2006; 8:220–220.
6. Kidd BL, Photiou A, Inglis JJ. The role of inflammatory mediators on nociception and pain in arthritis. Novartis Found Symp 2004; 260:122–133; discussion 133–138, 277–279.
7. Kidd BL, Urban LA. Mechanisms of inflammatory pain. Br J Anaesth 2001; 87:3–11.
8. Kulkarni B, Bentley DE, Elliott R, et al. Arthritic pain is processed in brain areas concerned with emotions and fear. Arthritis Rheum 2007; 56:1345–1354.
9. Baliki MN, Geha PY, Jabakhanji R, et al. A preliminary fMRI study of analgesic treatment in chronic back pain and knee osteoarthritis. Mol Pain 2008; 4:47.
10. Gwilym SE, Filippini N, Douaud G, et al. Thalamic atrophy associated with painful osteoarthritis of the hip is reversible after arthroplasty: a longitudinal voxel-based morphometric study. Arthritis Rheum 2010; 62:2930–2940.
11. Gwilym SE, Keltner JR, Warnaby CE, et al. Psychophysical and functional imaging evidence supporting the presence of central sensitization in a cohort of osteoarthritis patients. Arthritis Rheum 2009; 61:1226–1234.
12. Rogawski MA, Loscher W. The neurobiology of antiepileptic drugs for the treatment of nonepileptic conditions. Nat Med 2004; 10:685–692.
13. Onghena P, Van Houdenhove B. Antidepressant-induced analgesia in chronic non-malignant pain: a meta-analysis of 39 placebo-controlled studies. Pain 1992; 49:205–219.
14. Hauser W, Bernardy K, Uçeyler N, Sommer C. Treatment of fibromyalgia syndrome with gabapentin and pregabalin—a meta-analysis of randomized controlled trials. Pain 2009; 145:69–81.

15. Tzellos, TG, Toulis KA, Goulis DG, et al. Gabapentin and pregabalin in the treatment of fibromyalgia: a systematic review and a meta-analysis. J Clin Pharm Ther 2010; 35:639–656.

16. Rahman W, Bauer CS, Bannister K, et al. Descending serotonergic facilitation and the antinociceptive effects of pregabalin in a rat model of osteoarthritic pain. Mol Pain 2009; 5:45.

17. Jaffe M, Iacobelis D, Young JP, et al. Post-hoc results show beneficial effects of pregabalin in patients with osteoarthritis of the hip. Arthritis Rheum 2000; 43:S337.

18. Romano CL, Romanò D, Bonora C, Mineo G. Pregabalin, celecoxib, and their combination for treatment of chronic low-back pain. J Orthop Traumatol 2009; 10:185–191.

19. Sacre S, Medghalchi M, Gregory B, et al. Fluoxetine and citalopram exhibit potent antiinflammatory activity in human and murine models of rheumatoid arthritis and inhibit toll-like receptors. Arthritis Rheum 2010; 62:683–693.

20. Perrot S, Javier RM, Marty M, et al. Is there any evidence to support the use of anti-depressants in painful rheumatological conditions? Systematic review of pharmacological and clinical studies. Rheumatology 2008; 47:1117–1123.

21. Chan HN, Fam J, Ng BY. Use of antidepressants in the treatment of chronic pain. Ann Acad Med Singapore 2009; 38:974–979.

22. Jung AC, Staiger T, Sullivan M. The efficacy of selective serotonin reuptake inhibitors for the management of chronic pain. J Gen Intern Med 1997; 12:384–389.

23. Salerno SM, Browning R, Jackson JL. The effect of antidepressant treatment on chronic back pain: a meta-analysis. Arch Intern Med 2002; 162:19–24.

24. Chappell AS, Littlejohn G, Kajdasz DK, et al. A 1-year safety and efficacy study of duloxetine in patients with fibromyalgia. Clin J Pain 2009; 25:365–375.

25. Chwieduk CM, McCormack PL. Milnacipran: in fibromyalgia. Drugs 2010; 70:99–108.

26. Arnold LM, Lu Y, Crofford LJ, et al. A double-blind, multicenter trial comparing duloxetine with placebo in the treatment of fibromyalgia patients with or without major depressive disorder. Arthritis Rheum 2004; 50:2974–2984.

27. Arnold LM, Rosen A, Pritchett YL, et al. A randomized, double-blind, placebo-controlled trial of duloxetine in the treatment of women with fibromyalgia with or without major depressive disorder. Pain 2005; 119:5–15.

28. Clauw DJ, Mease P, Palmer RH, et al. Milnacipran for the treatment of fibromyalgia in adults: a 15-week, multicenter, randomized, double-blind, placebo-controlled, multiple-dose clinical trial. Clin Ther 2008; 30:1988–2004. [Erratum in Clin Ther. 2009 Feb;31:446]

29. Gendreau RM, Thorn MD, Gendreau JF, et al. Efficacy of milnacipran in patients with fibromyalgia. J Rheumatol 2005; 32:1975–1985.

30. Goldenberg DL, Clauw DJ, Palmer RH, et al. Durability of therapeutic response to milnacipran treatment for fibromyalgia. Results of a randomized, double-blind, monotherapy 6-month extension study. Pain Med 2010; 11:180–194.

31. Arnold LM, Clauw D, Wang F, et al. Flexible dosed duloxetine in the treatment of fibromyalgia: a randomized, double-blind, placebo-controlled trial. J Rheumatol 2010; 37:2578–2786.

32. Pertwee RG. Cannabinoid receptors and pain. Prog Neurobiol 2001; 63:569–611.

33. Swift W, Gates P, Dillon P. Survey of Australians using cannabis for medical purposes. Harm Reduct J 2005; 2:18.

34. Ware MA, Adams H, Guy GW. The medicinal use of cannabis in the UK: results of a nationwide survey. Int J Clin Pract 2005; 59:291–295.

35. Ware MA, Gamsa A, Persson J, Fitzcharles MA. Cannabis for chronic pain: case series and implications for clinicians. Pain Res Manag 2002; 7:95–99.

36. Blake DR, Robson P, Ho M, et al. Preliminary assessment of the efficacy, tolerability and safety of a cannabis-based medicine (Sativex) in the treatment of pain caused by rheumatoid arthritis. Rheumatology 2006; 45:50–52.

37. Ware MA, Fitzcharles MA, Joseph L, Shir Y. The effects of nabilone on sleep in fibromyalgia: results of a randomized controlled trial. Anesth Analg 2010; 110:604–610.

38. Skrabek RQ, Galimova L, Ethans K, Perry D. Nabilone for the treatment of pain in fibromyalgia. J Pain 2008; 9:164–173.

39. Aggarwal SK, Carter GT, Sullivan MD, et al. Characteristics of patients with chronic pain accessing treatment with medical cannabis in Washington State. J Opioid Manag 2009; 5:257–286.

40. Fiz J, Durán M, Capellà D, et al. Cannabis use in patients with fibromyalgia: effect on symptoms relief and health-related quality of life. PLoS One 2011; 6:e18440.

41. Kung T, Hochman J, Sun Y, et al. Efficacy and safety of cannabinoids for pain in musculoskeletal diseases: a systematic review and meta-analysis. J Rheumatol 2011; 38:1171.

42. Lynch ME, Clark AJ, Sawynok J, Sullivan MJ. Topical amitriptyline and ketamine in neuropathic pain syndromes: an open-label study. J Pain 2005; 6:644–649.

43. Bookman AA, Williams KS, Shainhouse JZ. Effect of a topical diclofenac solution for relieving symptoms of primary osteoarthritis of the knee: a randomized controlled trial. CMAJ 2004; 171:333–338.

44. Mason L, Moore RA, Edwards JE, et al. Topical NSAIDs for chronic musculoskeletal pain: systematic review and meta-analysis. BMC Musculoskelet Disord 2004; 5:28–28.

45. Mason L, Moore RA, Derry S, et al. Systematic review of efficacy of topical rubefacients containing salicylates for the treatment of acute and chronic pain. BMJ 2004; 328:995–995.

46. Harvey WF, Hunter DJ. The role of analgesics and intra-articular injections in disease management. Rheum Dis Clin N Am 2008; 34:777–788.

47. Khan MA, Gerner P, Kuo Wang G. Amitriptyline for prolonged cutaneous analgesia in the rat. Anesthesiology 2002; 96:109–116.

48. Sawynok J. Topical and peripherally acting analgesics. Pharmacol Rev 2003; 55:1–20.

49. Dominkus M, Nicolakis M, Kotz R, et al. Comparison of tissue and plasma levels of ibuprofen after oral and topical administration. Arzneimittelforschung 1996; 46:1138–1143.

50. Heyneman CA, Lawless-Liday C, Wall GC. Oral versus topical NSAIDs in rheumatic diseases: a comparison. Drugs 2000; 60:555–574.

51. Haroutiunian S, Drennan DA, Lipman AG. Topical NSAID therapy for musculoskeletal pain. Pain Med 2010; 11:535–549.

52. Lin J, Zhang W, Jones A, Doherty M. Efficacy of topical non-steroidal anti-inflammatory drugs in the treatment of osteoarthritis: meta-analysis of randomised controlled trials. BMJ 2004; 329:324.

53. Coombes BK, Bisset L, Vicenzino B. Efficacy and safety of corticosteroid injections and other injections for management of tendinopathy: a systematic review of randomised controlled trials. Lancet 2010; 376:1751–1767.

54. Bellamy N, Campbell J, Robinson V, et al. Intraarticular corticosteroid for treatment of osteoarthritis of the knee. Cochrane Database of Syst Rev 2006 Apr 19;(2):CD005328.

55. Creamer P. Intra-articular corticosteroid treatment in osteoarthritis. Curr Opin Rheum 1999; 11:417–421.

56. Gaujoux-Viala C, Dougados M, Gossec L. Efficacy and safety of steroid injections for shoulder and elbow tendonitis: a meta-analysis of randomised controlled trials. Ann Rheumatic Dis 2009; 68:1843–1849.

57. Bellamy N, Campbell J, Robinson V, et al. Viscosupplementation for the treatment of osteoarthritis of the knee. Cochrane Database Syst Rev 2006 Apr 19;(2):CD005321.

58. Reichenbach S, Blank S, Rutjes AW, et al. Hylan versus hyaluronic acid for osteoarthritis of the knee: a systematic review and meta-analysis. Arthritis Rheum 2007; 57:1410–1418.

59. Brzusek D, Petron D. Treating knee osteoarthritis with intra-articular hyaluronans. Curr Med Res Opin 2008; 24:3307–3322.

60. Boisset M, Fitzcharles MA. Alternative medicine use by rheumatology patients in a universal health care setting. J Rheumatol 1994; 21:148–152.

61. Ernst E. Complementary treatments in rheumatic diseases. Rheum Dis Clin N Am 2008; 34:455–467.

62. Kikuchi M, Matsuura K, Matsumoto Y, et al. Bibliographical investigation of complementary alternative medicines for osteoarthritis and rheumatoid arthritis. Geriatr Gerontol Int 2009; 9:29–40.

63. Ernst E. Musculoskeletal conditions and complementary/alternative medicine. Best Pract Res Clin Rheumatol 2004; 18:539–556.

64. Long L, Soeken K, Ernst E. Herbal medicines for the treatment of osteoarthritis: a systematic review. Rheumatology 2001; 40:779–793.

65. Goldberg RJ, Katz J. A meta-analysis of the analgesic effects of omega-3 polyunsaturated fatty acid supplementation for inflammatory joint pain. Pain 2007; 129:210–223.

66. Wandel S, Jüni P, Tendal B, et al. Effects of glucosamine, chondroitin, or placebo in patients with osteoarthritis of hip or knee: network meta-analysis. BMJ 2010; 341:c4675.

67. Holman AJ, Myers RR. A randomized, double-blind, placebo-controlled trial of pramipexole, a dopamine agonist, in patients with fibromyalgia receiving concomitant medications. Arthritis Rheum 2005; 52:2495–505.

68. Fitzgibbon EJ, Hall P, Schroder C, et al. Low dose ketamine as an analgesic adjuvant in difficult pain syndromes: a strategy for conversion from parenteral to oral ketamine. J Pain Symptom Manage 2002; 23:165–170.

69. Vergne-Salle P, Dufauret-Lombard C, Bonnet C, et al. A randomised, double-blind, placebo-controlled trial of dolasetron, a 5-hydroxytryptamine 3 receptor antagonist, in patients with fibromyalgia. Eur J Pain 2010; 15:509–14.

Chapter 9.4

Acute Postoperative Pain

Pierre Beaulieu

Introduction

The treatment of acute postoperative pain is an important healthcare issue [50]. It has been estimated that 234 million major surgical procedures are undertaken every year worldwide [49]. Many advances have been made in the pathophysiology of postoperative pain, and innovations in both analgesic agents and techniques for provision of analgesia have been developed. However, the management of acute postoperative pain is a real challenge, and even recently specialists in the field stated that there is still a long way to go [8]. The American Society of Anesthesiologists [1] has just published their guidelines for acute pain management in the perioperative setting. The purpose of these guidelines is to facilitate the safety and effectiveness of acute pain management, to reduce the risk of adverse outcomes, and to maintain the patient's functional abilities. Acute pain services must be established, and, most importantly, the development of educational programs for all persons involved in the care of surgical patients is crucial [8]. Finally, it has now been recognized that one of 10 surgical patients will develop chronic postoperative pain that constitutes a distressing healthcare problem and reduces quality of life [28]. A recent study has identified strong predictors for patients at risk for acute severe postoperative pain [46].

Pathophysiology of postoperative pain

The etiology and treatment of pain produced by surgery are different from other clinical pain conditions [11]. After in vivo neurophysiology experiments using the rat plantar incision [10], spontaneous activity in nociceptive pathways and guarding pain were reported after incision. This postoperative model indicates that different tissues have unique responses to incision: reducing the amount of deep tissue injury decreases pain at rest and opioid consumption, whereas varying the magnitude of the skin incision did not affect pain at rest or opioid use [11]. Furthermore, basic science data indicate that early after surgery, primary afferent activation and peripheral sensitization are profound when patients' postoperative pain is greatest. In addition, central sensitization likely contributes to referred pain and secondary hyperalgesia and perhaps to chronic posttraumatic pain [9].

In general, pain at rest resolves within the first week after surgery. Pain with activities, such as coughing or walking, is severe during the first 2 to 3 days then moderate or severe for many days or even weeks later.

Management of postoperative pain

The optimal management of postoperative pain is important, not only for humanitarian reasons (to decrease pain suffering immediately after surgery) but also because substandard acute pain management has far reaching consequences for the quality of life and consumption of healthcare resources for a large number of patients undergoing surgical procedures [8]. Many factors can influence the perception of postoperative pain (Table 9.4.1) [38].

General management: acute pain service

Acute pain management services evolved in response to the desire for improved management of postoperative pain. The concept of a collaborative, interdisciplinary approach to managing postoperative pain, which included formal education and the facilitation of clinical research in postoperative pain, was introduced in 1988 [41]. Nowadays, 90% of academic institutions have implemented a multidisciplinary team or acute pain service [7].

Table 9.4.1 Variables That May Affect Postoperative Pain Perception (from [38])
Demographic
• Age
• Gender
Sociocultural
• Ethnicity
• Educational level
• Income
• Family background
Psychological
• Anxiety
• Depression
• Vulnerability
• Locus of control
• Prior experience/expectations
• Cognitive components
Biological
• Genetics
• Concurrent medications
• Concurrent disease
• Anesthesia
• Surgery

Pharmacological management of postoperative pain

Multimodal analgesia

The definition and value of "multimodal" or "balanced analgesia" in postoperative pain treatment was proposed in 1993 by Kehlet and Dahl [27]. The American Society of Anesthesiologists [1] defines multimodal techniques for pain management as the administration of two or more drugs acting via different mechanisms to provide analgesia. This strategy seemed advantageous, inasmuch as analgesic power is enhanced together with an expected gain by reducing the risk of side effects compared with more intensive single-modality treatment. However, the optimal combination therapy needs to be evaluated regarding composition and duration for the various surgical procedures [27].

Today, multimodal analgesia includes the combined administration of acetaminophen, nonsteroidal anti-inflammatory drugs (NSAIDs), opioids, local anesthetics, and, more recently, anticonvulsant analgesics, ketamine, and possibly antidepressants. The idea behind multimodal analgesia is that combined drugs may have additive or even synergistic effects and at the same time allows the administration of smaller doses of the drugs with potentially more severe side effects. It is then hoped that using less opioids, for example, will be associated with less side effects [37]. Rather than simply focusing on the use of adjuvant analgesics for the management of postoperative pain, we also provide a brief overview of the multimodal analgesia, including use of acetaminophen, NSAIDs, and opioids.

Analgesics

Acetaminophen

The very low risk of acetaminophen therapy, with a highly favorable risk/benefit ratio, might justify a role for acetaminophen as a near-routine postoperative background analgesic as part of multimodal analgesia [35]. The maximal daily dose, when used for a short period of time such as postoperative pain, is 4 g in adults, 3 g in elderly or patients weighing less than 50 kg, and 60 mg/kg in children. An intravenous form now exists in most countries (Ofirmev in the United States, Perfalgan in Europe) that allows an administration even in patients nil by mouth as is often the case in the immediate postoperative period. The administration of intravenous acetaminophen reduces the use of other analgesics by 36%–50% [43]. Furthermore, the administration of acetaminophen with opioids was associated with a morphine-sparing effect of 20% for the first 24 hours, but without any difference in side-effect profile or patients' satisfaction [37, 42].

Nonsteroidal anti-inflammatory drugs

Selective cyclooxygenase-2 antagonists (coxibs) are as effective as standard NSAIDs in the management of postoperative pain. The administration of NSAIDs with morphine is associated with a morphine-sparing effect of 30%–50% and with a reduction in side effects: 30% less nausea and vomiting, 29% less sedation, but no effect on the incidence of pruritus, urinary retention, or respiratory depression [36, 37].

Nonsteroidal anti-inflammatory drugs and coxibs are associated with potentially serious side effects that restrain their utilization in the postoperative period. It is important to remember that the duration of treatment, the dose administered, and the age of the patient are crucial in producing unwanted effects: the longer the administration, the bigger the dose; and the older the patients are, the more deleterious effects are reported.

Nonsteroidal anti-inflammatory drugs, including coxibs, are contraindicated in patients with gastrointestinal, renal, cardiac (angina, cardiac failure), or cerebrovascular disease (transient ischemic events or stroke). Coxibs in particular should be used with caution in patients suffering from hypertension, dyslipidemia, diabetes, and in smokers. Finally, a short course of treatment at the lowest efficacious dose is highly recommended. An algorithm for the prescription of NSAIDs has been proposed for patients with gastrointestinal and cardiovascular problems [48].

Opioids

Opioids are the main treatment of moderate-to-severe postoperative pain in association with other analgesics. Spinal administration of opioids is discussed under "Local and Regional techniques". Systemic opioids are delivered through the oral, intravenous, subcutaneous/intramuscular, transmucosal, or nasal routes.

Side effects of opioids in the treatment of acute pain include the following: (1) Common: nausea and vomiting, respiratory depression, pruritus, urinary retention, ileus, sedation; (2) Less common: hallucinations, opioid-induced hyperalgesia (OIH); (3) Rare: physical dependence, addiction.

In the immediate postoperative period, opioids are administered either subcutaneously at regular intervals by a nurse or via a patient-controlled analgesia (PCA) device. When the patient can tolerate oral medications, opioids are administered orally if still needed. In a recent study, the intranasal route of administration of fentanyl has been developed. Its administration prevents gastrointestinal and hepatic presystemic elimination. It also allows fentanyl to enter the cerebrospinal fluid via the olfactorial mucosae, resulting in an immediate effect on the central nervous system. The onset time via this route is 6–8 minutes with a duration of analgesia of less than 1 hour. The intranasal route of administration of fentanyl has been used in the postoperative period with varying effects [24].

Patient-controlled analgesia

Patient-controlled analgesia administration is now the recommended technique for the administration of opioids postoperatively [20, 39]. Morphine is usually used, but hydromorphone or fentanyl are other options. After a loading dose, the bolus dose of the opioid and the lockout interval (minimal interval between two doses) must be set up for each patient.

Opioid-induced hyperalgesia

In the last few years, it has been observed that the administration of opioids can be associated with hyperalgesia (increased sensitivity to pain) rather than analgesia [3]. Indeed, opioid therapy, particularly in high doses, may cause heightened pain sensitivity and may aggravate preexisting pain. This paradoxical effect involves the N-methyl-D-aspartate (NMDA) receptors [45]. Therefore, the understanding of the pathophysiology of OIH has led to the administration of small doses of ketamine, a nonselective NMDA antagonist, for its prevention or treatment. The use of multimodal analgesia is also beneficial to try to avoid the development of OIH. It is important to note that tolerance and OIH are pharmacologically distinct phenomena and share the same net effect on dose requirements [3]. A more detailed discussion of OIH and the use of NMDA antagonists to treat postoperative pain can be found in Chapter 7.

Ketamine

Ketamine, a compound with analgesic and antihyperalgesic properties, has been shown to decrease postoperative pain and opioid requirements in adults [4, 40]. Routes of administration include intravenous, subcutaneous, epidural, transdermal, and intra-articular. At low subanesthetic doses (0.15–0.5 mg/kg), ketamine exerts a specific NMDA blockade effect and, hence, modulates central sensitization induced both by the incision and tissue damage and by perioperative analgesics such as opioids [47].

According to a meta-analysis [18] and a recent systematic review [29], ketamine administered intravenously during anesthesia in adults decreases postoperative pain intensity up to 48 hours, decreases total opioid consumption, and delays the time to first request of rescue analgesic. The greatest efficacy was found for thoracic, upper abdominal, and major orthopedic surgical subgroups. When ketamine was effective for pain, postoperative nausea and vomiting was less frequent in the ketamine group.

There is some evidence to show that perioperative administration of low-dose ketamine might modulate the expression of OIH or analgesic tolerance and that it reduces postoperative wound hyperalgesia after acute intraoperative opioid exposure [32].

Gabapentinoids

Multimodal treatment of postoperative pain using analgesic anticonvulsivants such as gabapentin or pregabalin (gabapentinoids) is becoming more common [16, 17]. The anti-hyperalgesic properties of gabapentin and pregabalin make them interesting analgesics to use in the perioperative period, to reduce pain and opioid consumption. Chapter 4 provides more information on pharmacological and pharmacokinetic properties of gabapentin and pregabalin. According to a recent systematic review of 11 randomized controlled trials, postoperative pain intensity is not reduced by pregabalin [51]. However, cumulative opioid consumption at 24 hours after surgery was significantly decreased with pregabalin (8.8 mg reduction for doses of pregabalin <300 mg and 13.4 mg for doses ≥300 mg). Pregabalin reduced opioid-related adverse effects such as vomiting, but the risk of visual disturbance was greater.

Another recent meta-analysis on pregabalin reported that the administration of 225–300 mg/day pregabalin during a short perioperative period provides additional analgesia in the short term but at the cost of additional adverse effects. Pregabalin increased the risk of dizziness or light-headedness and of visual disturbances, but it decreased the occurrence of postoperative nausea and vomiting [19].

For gabapentin, Clarke et al [13] reported that a single 600 mg dose given preoperatively or postoperatively does not reduce morphine consumption or pain scores in hospital or at 6 months after hip arthroplasty within the context of spinal anesthesia and a robust multimodal analgesia regimen. However, the same group reported that gabapentin decreases morphine consumption and improves functional recovery following total knee arthroplasty [14].

Therefore, further trials are needed to delineate the optimal dose, timing, and duration of pregabalin/gabapentin use following surgery and in which type of surgery they are effective. However, in acute pain setting, the current trend is to administer gabapentinoids 1 hour preoperatively ± 12 hours later. A dose of 600 mg (range, 300–1200 mg/day) of gabapentin or of 300 mg (range, 75–600 mg/day) of pregabalin is currently recommended [23].

Antidepressants

Antidepressant analgesics, in a similar manner to gabapentinoids, may have a role in the management of postoperative pain. However, only two studies are currently available [2, 25]. Therefore, their role in postoperative pain management and/or for the prevention of chronic pain after surgery is still not clear.

Local and regional techniques

Continuous nerve blockade is the only available medium- to long-term modality that blocks evoked pain. Decreased nausea and vomiting and increased patient satisfaction are seen with continuous peripheral nerve blocks, as well as possible improved rehabilitation and decreased incidence of postsurgery chronic pain syndromes.

The use of local anesthetics can be divided in different techniques and approaches: neuroaxial techniques, nerve or plexus blocks, incisional and intra-articular infiltrations (Table 9.4.2).

Neuroaxial techniques include mainly spinal and epidural anesthesia. Spinal opioids are usually administered with local anesthetics to allow surgery and to provide postoperative pain relief. Intrathecal morphine provides analgesia for approximately 24 hours after surgery. Patients should be monitored during this time for respiratory depression. Pruritus, nausea, and vomiting are common with spinal opioids. When compared with PCA with opioids, the epidural technique [21] offer some advantages (Table 9.4.3) [6].

With the development of echography, peripheral nerve or plexus blocks are often used to allow surgery but also to treat postoperative pain. The use of indwelling catheters will allow the infusion of local anesthetics for a few hours or days after surgery [26]. These techniques are used for upper and lower limb surgeries including orthopedic, general, and plastic surgery.

Continuous peripheral nerve blocks provide better pain control than opioids. Indeed, perineural catheters provide superior analgesia to opioids for all catheter locations and time periods. Nausea and vomiting, sedation, and pruritus all occurred more commonly with opioid analgesia, and a reduction in opioid use is noted with perineural analgesia [5].

The infiltration of the surgical wound with local anesthetics is now recommended in almost every patient [22]. It is not associated with wound dehiscence nor is it with the risk of skin infection. A perforated catheter may be inserted by the surgeon in the subcutaneous or subfascial space through which local anesthetics are infused postoperatively. The relief of postoperative pain by local anesthetic infiltration is effective in major abdominal and orthopedic surgery [15].

Table 9.4.2 Different Regional Techniques to Provide Postoperative Pain Relief

Neuroaxial blocks
• epidural
• spinal
• combined spinal/epidural
• caudal
Peripheral nerve and plexus blocks
• plexus blocks: brachial and lumbosacral
• proximal and distal nerves
• intercostal
• paravertebral
• transversus abdominis plane block
Incisional blocks: subcutaneous, subfascial
Intraarticular and intrabursal blocks

Intra-articular catheters are also inserted within major joints (hip, knee, shoulder) after surgery to allow the infusion of local anesthetics with good results compared with nerve blocks [31]. The use of liposomal formulations of local anesthetics prolongs analgesic duration and is an attractive new method of local anesthetic delivery [12].

Specific pain treatment

There is a need for the development of an evidence-based approach to reliable, comprehensive, individualized analgesic treatment. The number-needed-to-treat (NNT) of a particular analgesic can give a valuable overview of efficacy, but this concept is not necessarily applicable to all types of surgery.

Table 9.4.3 Comparison of Epidural Analgesia vs Opioid Patient-Controlled Analgesia (from [6])

	Epidural Analgesia (Local Anesthetics)	Opioid Patient-Controlled Analgesia
Pain control		
• at rest	+++	++
• on mobilization	++	±
Side effects		
• hypotension	−	+
• postoperative ileus	shortening	prolongation
• nausea/vomiting	−	++
• urinary retention	+	+
• sedation	−	+
Reduction in postoperative morbidity		
• cardiovascular	+	−
• respiratory	+	−
• nurses workload	+	+

Therefore, some groups have proposed that procedure-specific acute pain management guidelines may be helpful because the pain intensity and its consequences may be procedure-related [47]. Such procedure-specific guidelines are available from various sources, the main ones are as follows: (1) the PROSPECT (procedure specific pain treatment) Working Group (www.postoppain.org), a group of European anesthesiologists and surgeons; (2) the European Society of Regional Anaesthesia (ESRA) (www.esraeurope.org); and (3) the American Society of Anesthesiologists Task Force on Acute Pain Management with its updated report on Practice Guidelines for Acute Pain Management in the Perioperative Setting [1].

Chronic pain after surgery

The persistence of pain after surgical procedure or trauma has become a major focus of interest, and its prevention now represents a challenge as an indicator of quality of healthcare. Indeed, chronic pain after surgery has been a neglected topic until the last few years when it was realized that a wide variety of operations were associated with chronic pain syndromes. In order for pain to be classified as chronic postsurgical pain, the following criteria have to be established [34]: (1) pain develops after a surgical procedure; (2) pain is of at least 2 months duration; (3) other causes of pain should have been excluded (malignancy or chronic infection); and (4) pain is not due to an exacerbation of a preexistent condition. Acute postoperative pain is followed by persistent pain in 10%–50% of individuals after common operations, such as groin hernia repair, breast and thoracic surgery, leg amputation, and coronary artery bypass surgery; it can be severe in approximately 2%–10% of these patients [28]. The progression from acute to chronic postoperative pain has been recently reviewed [30, 44]. Several important risk factors involved in chronic pain development after tissue injury have been identified: preoperative pain and anxiety, repeat surgery, catastrophizing, female gender, surgical approach, moderate to severe acute postoperative pain, depression, radiation, or chemotherapy [30, 33]. In the future, the increasing understanding of genetic factors and the transitional mechanisms involved may reveal important clues to predict which patients will go on to develop chronic pain [44]. A combined scoring system based on age, sex, type and duration of surgery, extent of preoperative pain, obesity, and level of anxiety has been developed in an attempt to predict the severity of early postoperative pain. Large cohort studies are needed to validate the approach in individual procedures [28, 46, 50].

Future and conclusions

Preoperative pain is predictive of severe postoperative pain in 20% of the cases. Furthermore, severe postoperative pain, ie, pain not treated adequately, is associated with chronic pain in 10%–40% of patients. The best treatment is that of a balance between efficacy and acceptable side effects. Therefore, multimodal analgesia is the rule. Table 9.4.4 provides

Table 9.4.4 Summary of Nonopioid Drugs Used in the Postoperative Period

Drugs	Dose	Route of Administration	Frequency of Administration
Acetaminophen	650 mg	Oral	4 hourly
	1 g	Intravenous	6 hourly
Nonsteroidal anti-inflammatory drugs			
• naproxen	500 mg	Oral	12 hourly
• celecoxib	100 mg	Oral	12 hourly
Gabapentinoids			
• gabapentin	600 mg	Oral	1 h preoperatively
• pregabalin	300 mg	Oral	1 h preoperatively
Antidepressants*			
• venlafaxine	37.5 mg	Oral	Daily for 10 days postoperatively.
• duloxetine	60 mg	Oral	2 h preoperatively and at 24 h
Ketamine	0.15 mg/kg	Intravenous	Peroperatively
	10–15 µg/kg per min	Continuous intravenous infusion	Peroperatively
Local anesthetics	Maximal dose	Subcutaneous, subfascial, topical, epidural, perineural, intraarticular	4 hourly
• bupivacaine	2–3 mg/kg		
• levobupivacaine	2–3 mg/kg		
• ropivacaine	2 mg/kg		

*Based on one clinical study for each drug.

dosing guidelines for the most commonly used adjuvant analgesics in postoperative pain.

A hospital program for the management of postoperative pain should be in place in every center, offering patients analgesic options and a rehabilitation program based on the type of surgery and current evidence-based literature.

References

1. American Society of Anesthesiologists. Practice guidelines for acute pain management in the perioperative setting. Anesthesiology 2012; 116:248–273.
2. Amr YM, Yousef AA. Evaluation of efficacy of the perioperative administration of venlafaxine or gabapentin on acute and chronic postmastectomy pain. Clin J Pain 2010; 26:381–385.
3. Angst MS, Clark D. Opioid-induced hyperalgesia: a qualitative systematic review. Anesthesiology 2006; 104:570–587.
4. Beaulieu P. Non-opioid strategies for acute pain management. Can J Anesth 2007; 54:481–485.
5. Boezaart AP. Perineural infusion of local anesthetics. Anesthesiology 2006; 104:872–880.

6. Bonnet F, Marret E. Influence of anaesthetic and analgesic techniques on outcome after surgery. Br J Anaesth 2005; 95:52–58.

7. Breivik H, Curatolo M, Niemi G, et al. How to implement an acute postoperative pain service: an update. In: Breivik H, Shipley M, eds. *Pain—Best Practice and Research Compendium*. London: Elsevier; 2007. pp 255–270.

8. Breivik H, Stubhaug A. Management of acute postoperative pain: Still a long way to go! Pain 2008; 137:233–234.

9. Brennan TJ, Kehlet H. Preventive analgesia to reduce wound hyperalgesia and persistent postsurgical pain: not an easy path. Anesthesiology 2005; 103:681–683.

10. Brennan TJ, Vandermeulen EP, Gebhart GF. Characterization of a rat model of incisional pain. Pain 1996; 64:493–501.

11. Brennan TJ. Pathophysiology of postoperative pain. Pain 2011; 152: S33–S40.

12. Cereda CM, Brunetto GB, de Araujo DR, de Paula E. Liposomal formulations of prilocaine, lidocaine and mepivacaine prolong analgesic duration. Can J Anesth 2006; 53:1092–1097.

13. Clarke H, Pereira S, Kennedy D, et al. Adding gabapentin to a multimodal regimen does not reduce acute pain, opioid consumption or chronic pain after total hip arthroplasty. Acta Anaesthesiol Scand 2009; 53:1073–1083.

14. Clarke H, Pereira S, Kennedy D, et al. Gabapentin decreases morphine consumption and improves functional recovery following total knee arthroplasty. Pain Res Manag 2009; 14:217–222.

15. Dahl JB, Møiniche S. Relief of postoperative pain by local anaesthetic infiltration: Efficacy for major abdominal and orthopedic surgery. Pain 2009; 143:7–11.

16. Dauri M, Faria S, Gatti A, et al. Gabapentin and pregabalin for the acute post-operative pain management. A systematic-narrative review of the recent clinical evidences. Curr Drug Targets 2009; 10:716–733.

17. Durkin B, Page C, Glass P. Pregabalin for the treatment of postsurgical pain. Expert Opin Pharmacother 2010; 11:2751–2758.

18. Elia N, Tramer MR. Ketamine and postoperative pain: a quantitative systematic review of randomised trials. Pain 2005; 113:61–70.

19. Engelman E, Cateloy F. Efficacy and safety of perioperative pregabalin for post-operative pain: a meta-analysis of randomized-controlled trials. Acta Anaesthesiol Scand 2011; 55:927–943.

20. Franson HE. Postoperative patient-controlled analgesia in the pediatric population: a literature review. AANA J 2010; 78:374–378.

21. Freise H, Van Aken HK. Risks and benefits of thoracic epidural anaesthesia. Br J Anaesth 2011; 107:859–868.

22. Ganapathy S, Brookes J, Bourne R. Local infiltration analgesia. Anesthesiol Clin 2011; 29:329–342.

23. Gilron I. Gabapentin and pregabalin for chronic neuropathic and early postsurgical pain: current evidence and future directions. Curr Opin Anaesthesiol 2007; 20:456–472.

24. Hansen MS, Mathiesen O, Trautner S, Dahl JB. Intranasal fentanyl in the treatment of acute pain—a systematic review. Acta Anaesthesiol Scand 2012; 56:407–19.

25. Ho KY, Tay W, Yeo MC, et al. Duloxetine reduces morphine requirements after knee replacement surgery. Br J Anaesth 2010; 105:371–376.

26. Ilfeld BM. Continuous peripheral nerve blocks: a review of the published evidence. Anesth Analg 2011; 113:904–925.

27. Kehlet H, Dahl J. The value of "multimodal" or "balanced analgesia" in postoperative pain treatment. Anesth Analg 1993; T7:1048–1056.

28. Kehlet H, Jensen TS, Woolf CJ. Persistent postsurgical pain: risk factors and prevention. Lancet 2006; 367:1618–1625.

29. Laskowski K, Stirling A, McKay WP, Lim HJ. A systematic review of intravenous ketamine for postoperative analgesia. Can J Anaesth 2011; 58:911–923.

30. Lavand'homme P. The progression from acute to chronic pain. Curr Opin Anaesthesiol 2011; 24:545–550.

31. Lavelle W, Lavelle ED, Lavelle L. Intra-articular injections. Anesthesiol Clin 2007; 25:853–862.

32. Lee M, Silverman S, Hansen H, et al. A comprehensive review of opioid-induced hyperalgesia. Pain Physician 2011; 14:145–161.

33. Macintyre PE, Schug Sa, Scott DA, et al. *Acute Pain Management: Scientific Evidence*, 3rd edition, Australian and New Zealand College of Anaesthetists. Melbourne: 2010; www.fpm.anzca.edu.au/resources/books-and-publications/publications-1/Acute%20Pain%20-%20final%20version.pdf.

34. Macrae WA. Chronic post-surgical pain: 10 years on. Br J Anaesth 2008; 101:77–86.

35. Mallet C, Eschalier A. Pharmacology and mechanism of action of acetaminophen. In: *Pharmacology of Pain*. Beaulieu P, Lussier D, Porreca D, Dickenson AH, eds. Seattle: IASP Press; 2010: pp 65–85.

36. Marret E, Kurdi O, Zufferey P, Bonnet F. Effects of nonsteroidal anti-inflammatory drugs on patient-controlled analgesia morphine side effects: meta-analysis of randomized controlled trials. Anesthesiology 2005; 102:1249–1260.

37. Maund E, McDaid C, Rice S, et al. Paracetamol and selective and non-selective non-steroidal anti-inflammatory drugs for the reduction in morphine-related side-effects after major surgery: a systematic review. Br J Anaesth 2011; 106:292–27.

38. Nielsen PR, Rudin A, Werner MU. Prediction of postoperative pain. Curr Anaesth Crit Care 2007; 18:157–165.

39. Palmer PP, Miller RD. Current and developing methods of patient-controlled analgesia. Anesthesiol Clin 2010; 28:587–599.

40. Quibell R, Prommer EE, Mihalyo M, et al. Ketamine. J Pain Sympt Manag 2011; 41:640–649.

41. Ready LB, Oden R, Chadwick HS, et al. Development of an anesthesiology-based postoperative pain management service. Anesthesiology 1988; 68:100–106.

42. Remy C, Marret E, Bonnet F. Effects of acetaminophen on morphine side-effects and consumption after major surgery: meta-analysis of randomized controlled trials. Br J Anaesth 2005; 94:505–513.

43. Romsing J, Moiniche S, Dahl JB. Rectal and parenteral paracetamol, and paracetamol in combination with NSAIDs, for postoperative analgesia. Br J Anaesth 2002; 88:215–226.

44. Shipton EA. The transition from acute to chronic post surgical pain. Anaesth Intensive Care 2011; 39:824–836.

45. Simonnet G, Rivat C. Opioid-induced hyperalgesia: abnormal or normal pain? Neuroreport 2003; 14:1–7.

46. Sommer M, de Rijke JM, van Kleef M, et al. Predictors of acute postoperative pain after elective surgery. Clin J Pain 2010; 26:87–94.

47. Vadivelu N, Mitra S, Narayan D. Recent advances in postoperative pain management. Yale J Biol Med 2010; 83:11–25.

48. Vergne-Salle P, Beneytout JL. Targeting the cyclooxygenase pathway. In: *Pharmacology of Pain*. Beaulieu P, Lussier D, Porreca D, Dickenson AH, eds. Seattle: IASP Press; 2010: pp 43–64.

49. Weiser TG, Regenbogen SE, Thompson KD, et al. An estimation of the global volume of surgery: a modelling strategy based on available data. Lancet 2008; 372:139–44.

50. Wu CL, Raja SN. Treatment of acute postoperative pain. Lancet 2011; 377:2215–2225.

51. Zhang J, Ho KY, Wang Y. Efficacy of pregabalin in acute postoperative pain: a meta-analysis. Br J Anaesth 2011; 106:454–462.

Chapter 10
Drug-Drug Interactions of Adjuvant Analgesics

David R. P. Guay

Introduction

Drugs can interact with other drugs, excipients in the dosage formulation, components of large-volume parenteral solutions, foodstuffs, nutrients, etc. For purposes of this chapter, only drug-drug interactions will be presented. Drug-drug interactions can affect the pharmacokinetics (ie, absorption, distribution, metabolism, and excretion) or pharmacodynamics (ie, responses good and bad) of one or both drugs involved. An adverse reaction may, in turn, result. The severity of drug-drug interactions is influenced by several factors including the therapeutic indices of the drugs (ie, the ratio of toxic to therapeutic concentrations or doses), age-related changes in physiology applicable to the mechanism of the interaction, drug doses, and, in some cases, pharmacogenetics. Pharmacogenetics, as applied to drug-drug interactions, centers around genetic-based differences in drug metabolism (eg, poor vs extensive metabolizers of specific cytochrome P450 isozymes). This chapter will present drug-drug interactions of adjuvant analgesics with other adjuvant analgesics or drugs of other classes.

Drug-Drug interactions involving prescription and over-the-counter medications

Tables 10.1 and 10.2 illustrate the most common and important drug-drug interactions occurring between two adjuvant analgesics (Table 10.1) or an adjuvant analgesic with another class of analgesic (Table 10.2).

Serotonin toxicity

One of the most significant drug-drug interactions involving serotonergic medications involves potentiation of the effect of the neurotransmitter serotonin in the synapse. Table 10.3 illustrates drugs enhancing serotonergic activity [28]. Serotonergic analgesics in Table 10.3 have been italicized. The most acute manifestation of serotonin excess at the synapse is referred to as serotonin toxicity or serotonin syndrome. This is

Table 10.1 Interactions Between Diverse Adjuvant Analgesics

Adjuvant	Other Adjuvant	Interactions	Mechanism	Evidence	Recommendations
TCAs [1]	SSRIs, SNRIs	↑ serotonergic effects	• Additive serotonergic effects at synapse • Inhibition of TCA drug metabolism by SSRIs/SNRIs (inhibition of CYP450 isozymes 2D6, 1A2, 2C9, 2C19, 3A4. Note: range of number of isozymes inhibited and potency of inhibition vary between SSRIs) → ↑ TCA (parent +/− active metabolite) serum concentrations → serotonergic effects at synapse	Reported with • Amitriptyline + sertraline • Imipramine/desipramine + fluvoxamine • Clomipramine + fluvoxamine • TCAs + fluvoxamine • TCAs + venlafaxine	• Avoid this combination if possible • If must use a TCA, avoid clomipramine as it is the most serotonergic TCA • If must use a SSRI, use citalopram or escitalopram because these interact least with CYP450 isozymes
TCAs [1]	Phenytoin	↑ plasma phenytoin concentrations	Unknown	• Case report with imipramine • No interaction in case series with nortriptyline and amitriptyline	Use TCA other than imipramine
CBZ [2]	Valproate	• Variable effects on plasma CBZ concentrations • ↑ plasma CBZ epoxide concentrations • ↓ plasma valproate concentrations	• Valproate inhibits CBZ metabolism, displaces it from plasma protein binding sites, inhibits CBZ epoxide metabolism • CBZ induces valproate metabolism	• Pharmacokinetic studies	Careful monitoring of toxicity/loss of efficacy and therapeutic drug monitoring are necessary whenever regimen of either agent is altered

CBZ [2, 3]	Phenytoin	• ↓ plasma CBZ concentrations • Variable effect on plasma phenytoin concentrations	• Each induces the hepatic metabolism of the other • Compete for metabolic enzymes in the liver (substrate inhibitors) and thus function as "enzyme inhibitors"	• Pharmacokinetic studies	Careful monitoring of toxicity/loss of efficacy and therapeutic drug monitoring are necessary whenever regimen of either agent is altered
CBZ [2, 4]	Lamotrigine	• ↓ lamotrigine plasma concentration • ↑ CBZ epoxide plasma concentrations	• Lamotrigine impairs CBZ epoxide clearance • CBZ induces lamotrigine metabolism	• Case series • Pharmacokinetic studies	Careful monitoring of toxicity/loss of efficacy and therapeutic drug monitoring are necessary whenever regimen of either agent is altered
CBZ [1, 2, 5]	TCAs	• ↓ plasma TCA concentrations	• Induction of TCA CYP450-mediated metabolism by CBZ	• Therapeutic drug monitoring retrospective studies • Pharmacokinetic studies	• Avoid combination if possible. • Monitor carefully if CBZ regimen is changed. • May require therapeutic drug monitoring of both drugs. • Beware TCA toxicity if CBZ dose is reduced or CBZ therapy is stopped without a reduction in TCA dose.

(*continued*)

Table 10.1 Continued

Adjuvant	Other Adjuvant	Interactions	Mechanism	Evidence	Recommendations
Lamotrigine [6]	Phenytoin	• ↓ lamotrigine plasma concentrations	• Induction of lamotrigine metabolism by phenytoin	• Pharmacokinetic studies	• Dramatic ↓ lamotrigine concentration is unlikely • Following lamotrigine plasma concentrations during phenytoin dose titration and subsequent phenytoin dose adjustments is reasonable
TCA [7]	Venlafaxine Duloxetine	• ↑ plasma TCA concentrations	• Venlafaxine- or duloxetine-associated inhibition of CYP2D6-mediated metabolism of TCA. Should preferentially affect desipramine, imipramine, amitriptyline and doxepin.	• Pharmacokinetic studies	• Avoid the combination by substituting an SSRI with minimal CYP450 isozyme 2D6—inhibiting potential (eg, citalopram) for venlafaxine/duloxetine and/or substituting a TCA not dependent on CYP450 isozyme 2D6 for its metabolism (eg, nortriptyline).

Abbreviations: CBZ, carbamazepine; SNRIs, serotonin norepinephrine reuptake inhibitors; SSRIs, selective serotonin reuptake inhibitors; TCAs, tricyclic antidepressants.

Table 10.2 Interactions Between Adjuvant Analgesics and Other Analgesics

Adjuvant	Other Analgesic	Interactions	Mechanism	Evidence	Recommendations
Imipramine [8]	ASA	• ↑ adverse effects of imipramine, transient if adequate renal/hepatic function	ASA ↑unbound (free) plasma concentrations via plasma protein displacement	One case series	Transient effect, so monitor for ↑ adverse effects of imipramine at initiation of ASA
TCAs [9, 10]	NSAIDs	↑ risk of upper gastrointestinal bleeding	Unknown. Possible additive/synergistic antiplatelet effects of TCAs and NSAIDs	• Population-based, case-cohort study reported ↑ bleeding risk; however, lower than with SSRI-NSAID combinations • Another study did not observe interaction	• Replace TCA by another antidepressant with minimal or no serotonergic activity or • Replace NSAID by nonacetylated salicylate, celecoxib or acetaminophen • If must use a TCA and NSAID, use desipramine, trimipramine, or nortriptyline because these are minimally serotonergic
CBZ [11]	Methadone	• ↓ methadone plasma concentrations • Withdrawal of CBZ → ↑ methadone plasma concentration unless methadone dose is decreased	• CBZ induces hepatic metabolism of methadone • Removal of CBZ causes deinduction of methadone metabolism back to baseline level	• Case series of patients on methadone maintenance therapy who experienced opioid withdrawal symptoms after introduction of CBZ • Case report of methadone-associated respiratory depression after discontinuation of CBZ	• Avoid combination if possible • If not possible, careful monitoring when dose of CBZ is altered • Monitor for necessary adjustment of methadone dose after CBZ discontinuation

(continued)

Table 10.2 Continued

Adjuvant	Other Analgesic	Interactions	Mechanism	Evidence	Recommendations
CBZ [12]	Codeine	• ↑ production of active codeine metabolite, normorphine	• ↑ N-demethylation pathways of codeine by hepatic enzyme-inducing effects of CBZ → ↑ urinary excretion of norcodeine while urinary excretion of normorphine is unchanged	• Case series of epileptic patients	Clinical relevance unknown
Lamotrigine [13]	Acetaminophen	• ↓ lamotrigine plasma concentrations with initiation of acetaminophen	• Unknown	• Pharmacokinetic studies in eight healthy volunteers	• Unclear clinical relevance • Likely clinically relevant only with chronic acetaminophen usage
Corticosteroids [14]	Phenytoin	• ↓ plasma corticosteroid and phenytoin concentrations	• Phenytoin-associated enhancement of corticosteroid metabolism (eg, 6–hydroxylation) and • Corticosteroid-associated enhancement of phenytoin metabolism (primarily seen with dexamethasone).	• Case series • Pharmacokinetic studies	• Avoid this combination if possible • May need to ↑ corticosteroid dose by ≥2-fold and phenytoin dose, too, to compensate for this interaction

Prednisone	NSAIDs	• ↑ incidence/severity of NSAID-associated and/or corticosteroid-associated peptic ulcer disease, gastritis, etc	• Additive gastrointestinal mucosal injury	• Theoretical interaction. Few data available	• Use local corticosteroids where applicable (topical skin, nasal cavity, rectum, lung, eye) and/or • Add peptic ulcer disease prophylaxis (misoprostol 400–800 mcg/day, standard-dose proton pump inhibitor, double-dose histamine 2 blocker)
Duloxetine Venlafaxine SSRIs [9, 10, 15, 16]	NSAIDs	• ↑ risk of upper gastrointestinal bleeding	• Unknown • Possibly additive platelet function inhibition	• Large population-based, cohort study • Nested case-control study • Meta-analysis of observational studies	• Such combination therapy should be avoided • If cannot be avoided, replace one or both of the interacting agents: NSAID with acetaminophen or celecoxib and/or SSRI/SNRI with noradrenergic TCA (desipramine, nortriptyline)
Bisphosphonates (oral only) [17, 18]	NSAIDs	• ↑ risk of gastric ulcer	• Additive irritative effects on gastric mucosa	• Open-label study in 26 healthy volunteers • Retrospective case-control study did not find interaction	• Use alternatives for 1 or both agents. • Monitor for gastrointestinal adverse effects. • No data supporting efficacy of misoprostol, proton pump inhibitor, and histamine H2 blocker prophylaxis with this combination. However, the American Gastroenterological Association does recommend prophylaxis with one of these agents if oral bisphophonate-NSAID therapy must be used concurrently.

(*continued*)

Table 10.2 Continued

Adjuvant	Other Analgesic	Interactions	Mechanism	Evidence	Recommendations
Serotonergic antidepressant (SSRIs, venlafaxine, mirtazapine, trazodone, imipramine, clomipramine)	Tramadol [19–23] Tapentadol (possibly same liabilities as tramadol) [24] Methadone [25, 26]	• Precipitation of serotonin syndrome	• Additive effects on serotonergic neurotransmission	• Several case reports, including lethal interaction	Substitute a minimal or nonserotonergic antidepressant and/or nonserotonergic analgesic.
Paroxetine and other inhibitors of CYP2D6 [27]	Tramadol	• ↓ tramadol efficacy	• ↓ generation of active O-desmethyl metabolite	• pharmacokinetic studies	Use antidepressant that does not inhibit CYP2D6

Abbreviations: ASA, aspirin; CBZ, carbamazepine; NSAIDs, nonsteroidal anti-inflammatory drugs; SNRIs, serotonin norepinephrine reuptake inhibitors; SSRIs, selective serotonin reuptake inhibitors; TCA, tricyclic antidepressants.

Table 10.3 Drugs Which Increase Serotonergic Activity

Inhibition of 5-HT Release[a]	Inhibition of 5-HT Metabolism	Stimulation of Postsynaptic Receptor Pathway	Stimulation of 5-HT Release[b]	Stimulation of 5-HT Synthesis
SSRIs	*MAOIs*	Carbamazepine	Amphetamine	5-Hydroxy tryptophan
Fluoxetine	Moclobemide	Lithium	MDMA (ecstacy)	L-tryptophan
Paroxetine	Selegiline	5-HT$_1$ agonists	Fenfluramine	
Sertraline	Rasagiline[c]	Sumatriptan	Cocaine	
Fluvoxamine	Tranylcypromine		*MAOIs*	
Citalopram	Phenelzine		Moclobemide	
SNRIs	St. John's Wort		Selegiline	
Venlafaxine			Rasagiline[c]	
Duloxetine			Tranylcypromine	
TCAs			Phenelzine	
Amitriptyline				
Imipramine				
Clomipramine				
Doxepin				
Desipramine				
Other ADs				
Trazodone				
Nefazodone				
Opioids				
Tramadol				
Tapentadol[c]				
Meperidine				
Methadone				
Fentanyl[d]				
Dextromethorphan				

(continued)

Table 10.3 Continued				
Inhibition of 5-HT Release[a]	Inhibition of 5-HT Metabolism	Stimulation of Postsynaptic Receptor Pathway	Stimulation of 5-HT Release[b]	Stimulation of 5-HT Synthesis
Others				
Amphetamine				
Cocaine				
St. John's Wort				

Abbreviations: ADs, antidepressants; 5-HT, serotonin; MAOIs, monoamine oxidase inhibitors; MDMA, methylenedioxymethamphetamine; SSRI, selective serotonin reuptake inhibitor; SNRIs, serotonin norepinephrine reuptake inhibitors; TCAs, tricyclic antidepressants.

[a]From synapse.
[b]From nerve terminals.
[c]Presumably similar to immediately preceding agent based on structural and pharmacological similarities.
[d]And congeners such as sufentanil and alfentanil.
[Modified from Ref. 28.]

a predictable consequence of serotonergic excess in the central nervous system, resulting from the administration of serotonin-active drugs. Seven mechanisms can produce serotonin syndrome: increased serotonin synthesis, increased serotonin release, inhibition of the serotonin reuptake transporter, inhibition of the metabolism of serotonin in the synaptic cleft (ie, inhibition of monoamine oxidase), direct stimulation of serotonin receptors, increased sensitivity of the postsynaptic response, and (possibly) decreased dopaminergic activity (with only a modest concurrent increase in serotonin activity) [28].

Although many drugs have been implicated in the precipitation of serotonin syndrome, the majority of cases involve selective serotonin reuptake inhibitors and serotonin norepinephrine reuptake inhibitors. Although from an analgesic point of view, only venlafaxine and duloxetine are represented in these two classes. The tricyclic antidepressants are the next most important class of serotonin-active compounds, which are also analgesic compounds. In addition, the serotonergic opioids—especially tramadol and methadone—are becoming more important contributors to serotonin toxicity. From a pharmacodynamic perspective, administering two serotonergic drugs at the same time may lead to additive or synergistic serotonergic effects, resulting in serotonin toxicity [28].

In addition to the pharmacodynamic mechanisms that cause these agents to produce serotonin excess, one must add pharmacokinetic factors, which may contribute not only to the onset but also to the intensity of serotonin toxicity. This is why agents with long-terminal disposition half-lives such as fluoxetine and its active metabolite norfluoxetine can produce very long periods of risk, even after drug cessation, of serotonin excess should another serotonin-active drug be started. This is also why the addition of a drug inhibiting the metabolism of a serotonin-active drug may actually precipitate serotonin toxicity. There are many agents that can inhibit one or more isozymes of the cytochrome P450 family of drug-metabolizing enzymes. Addition of one of these "enzyme inhibitors" will lead to a reduction in metabolism of the other (serotonergic) drug, causing drug accumulation until serotonin toxicity supervenes. In other cases, enzyme inhibition will lead to a reduction in analgesic effect if it results in reduced generation of an active metabolite (eg, tramadol, codeine). In other cases, the addition of an "enzyme stimulant" may lead to enhanced drug metabolism and a reduction in drug (ie, analgesic) response [28]. More details regarding serotonin toxicity are available in the relevant sections of Tables 10.1 and 10.2.

A survey was conducted in Australia of deaths from 2002 to 2008, wherein one or more of the following serotonergic drugs were found at autopsy: tramadol, venlafaxine, fluoxetine, sertraline, citalopram, paroxetine, and MDMA (ecstasy). Although 1123 such deaths were found, in 28 cases there were signs or symptoms antemortem, which was suggestive of serotonin syndrome and believed to have contributed to the subjects' death. In 11 cases, two or more potential analgesic agents were found. Tramadol and venlafaxine were involved in six cases each. Among the six venlafaxine recipients, five and one subject had venlafaxine plus an opioid (tramadol in one, methadone in four) and venlafaxine plus a tricyclic antidepressant (amitriptyline) present, respectively. In addition, the relative prevalences of these serotonergic agents in the 1123 cases were calculated by adjusting for annual drug consumption of these agents in Australia over the 2002–2008 data collection period. Tramadol scored 10.15 followed by ecstasy (4.57), fluoxetine (3.02), and the remainder (≤1.47). The data from this report substantiate the lethal potential for serotonergic combinations, especially those involving either tramadol or venlafaxine [19].

There are striking similarities between tramadol and venlafaxine that may explain the findings just described. First, the structural similarities are great: each has methoxyphenyl, N,N-dimethylamino, and hydroxycyclohexyl groups (groups may assume near-superimposable intermolecular orientations). Second, they have the same prominent adverse effects (nausea, headache, dizziness). Third, both inhibit the reuptake of serotonin and norepinephrine. Fourth, both undergo enantioselective metabolism via CYP450 isozyme 2D6. Finally, both are metabolized to active desmethyl metabolites.

Drug-drug interactions involving herbals or complementary and alternative medications

An area of ever-increasing interest is the interaction of drugs with herbal or complementary and alternative medications (CAMs). A major problem with the latter medications is the lack of regulatory oversight with respect to their pharmacology/pharmacokinetics/pharmacodynamics, which, in turn,

CHAPTER 10 Drug-drug Interactions

Table 10.4 Interactions Between Herbals and Analgesics

Herbal	Analgesic	Interactions	Mechanism	Evidence	Recommendations
Garlic [29]	Acetaminophen	↑ exposure to acetaminophen and its glucuronide metabolite	Unknown	Pharmacokinetic study	Unlikely to be clinically significant
Garlic [30]	NSAIDs	Possible ↑ bleeding risk	Garlic ↓ platelet aggregation as do NSAIDs	Theoretical assumption without clinical data of effect of combination of garlic-NSAIDs on bleeding risk	Likely clinically relevant only with excessive doses of garlic
Gingko [31]	Aspirin	No additive effects occur for the combination of ginkgo 300 mg daily and aspirin 325 mg daily over 2 weeks in terms of clotting time or platelet aggregation.		Randomized controlled trial	No interaction
Gingko [32]	Ibuprofen	Possible ↑ bleeding risk		One case report of fatal intracerebral bleed	No clear evidence of interaction
Gingko [33]	Anticonvulsants metabolised by CYP2C19	↓ plasma concentrations of anticonvulsants	CYP2C19 induction by gingko	One case report of fatal seizure in one patient on stable doses of phenytoin and valproate who started gingko	No clear evidence of interaction
St. John's Wort [34]	Amitriptyline	↓ systemic exposure to amitriptyline and its active metabolite nortriptyline	Induction of CYP3A4 and/or P-gp by St. John's Wort	Crossover trial evaluating plasma concentrations of amitriptyline and nortriptyline with/without concurrent St. John's Wort	Monitor therapeutic response
St. John's Wort [35]	Venlafaxine	Precipitation of serotonin syndrome	Unknown. No causality established.	Case report of serotonin syndrome in patient on venlafaxine who started St. John's Wort, resolved after discontinuation	No clear interaction or causality
St. John's Wort [36]	Methadone	↓ plasma concentrations of methadone	Induction of CYP3A4 and/or P-gp by St. John's Wort	Pharmacokinetic study in 4 patients	Monitor therapeutic response. Beware opioid withdrawal signs/symptoms

Abbreviations: NSAIDs, nonsteroidal anti-inflammatory drugs; P-gp, P-glycoprotein.

may not allow the practitioner to make predictions of drug-drug interaction potential. It is only through the case report mechanism that drug-drug interactions may come to light. In addition, manufacturers of these products are generally not sufficiently capitalized to investigate the mechanisms and epidemiology of drug-drug interactions with their herbal/CAM products. As one can see from Table 10.4, some of these drug-drug interactions can have clinically important effects [29–36].

Summary

Of all drug-drug interactions involving adjuvant analgesics reviewed in Tables 10.1, 10.2, and 10.4, only a few are likely to be of high potential clinical significance. These include the following:

- tricyclic antidepressants/venlafaxine/duloxetine/oral bisphosphonates + nonsteroidal anti-inflammatory drugs: increased risk of upper gastrointestinal bleeding due to additive antiplatelet effects
- oral bisphosphonates + multivalent cations (eg, calcium, magnesium, iron, aluminium): malabsorption of biphosphonate
- two or more drug combinations of serotonergic agents, including serotonergic analgesics such as tricyclic antidepressants, venlafaxine, duloxetine, and serotonergic opioids (tramadol/tapentadol, methadone, meperidine, fentanyl and its congeners): risk of serotonin syndrome
- carbamazepine or phenytoin + other analgesics/agents metabolized by CYP 450 hepatic enzymes: variable plasma concentrations when one drug is initiated or discontinued
- CYP450 isozyme 2D6 inhibitors + tramadol: decreased efficacy of tramadol

When adding an adjuvant analgesic to a pharmaceutical regimen, one should always take into account potential drug-drug interactions, especially the most clinically relevant, to avoid increased toxicity or decreased efficacy.

References

1. Gilman PK. Tricyclic antidepressant pharmacology and therapeutics: drug interactions updated. Br J Pharmacol 2007; 151:737–748.

2. Ramsey RE, McManus DQ, Gutterman A, et al. Carbamazepine metabolism in humans: effect of concurrent anticonvulsant therapy. Ther Drug Monit 1990; 12:235–241.

3. Browne TR, Szabo GK, Evans JE, et al. Carbamazepine increases phenytoin serum concentration and reduces phenytoin clearance. Neurology 1988; 38:1146–1150.

4. Malminiemi K, Keranen T, Kerrtula T, et al. Effects of short-term lamotrigine treatment on pharmacokinetics of carbamazepine. Int J Clin Pharmacol Ther 2000; 38:540–545.

5. Leinonen E, Lillsunde P, Laukkanen V, Ylitalo P. Effects of carbamazepine on serum antidepressant concentrations in psychiatric patients. J Clin Psychopharmacol 1991; 11:313–318.

6. Wolf P. Lamotrigine: preliminary clinical observations on pharmacokinetics and interactions with traditional antiepileptic drugs. J Epilepsy 1992; 5:73–79.

7. Patroneva A, Connolly SM, Fatato P, et al. An assessment of drug-drug interactions: the effect of desvenlafaxine and duloxetine on the pharmacokinetics of the CYP 2D6 probe desipramine in healthy subjects. Drug Metab Dispos 2008; 36:2484–2491.

8. Juarez-Olguin H, Jung-Cook H, Flores-Perez J, Asseff IL. Clinical evidence of an interaction between imipramine and acetylsalicylic acid on protein binding in depressed patients. Clin Neuropharmacol 2002; 25:32–36.

9. Dalton SO, Johansen C, Mellemkjaer L, et al. Use of selective serotonin reuptake inhibitors and risk of upper gastrointestinal tract bleeding: a population-based cohort study. Arch Intern Med 2003; 163:59–64.

10. De Abajo FJ, Garcia Rodriguez LA, Montero D. Association between selective serotonin reuptake inhibitors and upper gastrointestinal tract bleeding: population-based case-control study. BMJ 1999; 319:1106–1109.

11. Benitez-Rosario MA, Martin AS, Gomez-Ontanon E, Feria M. Methadone-induced respiratory depression after discontinuing carbamazepine administration. J Pain Symptom Manage 2006; 32:99–100.

12. Yue QY, Tomson T, Sauve J. Carbamazepine and cigarette smoking induce differentially the metabolism of codeine in man. Pharmacogenetics 1994; 4:193–198.

13. Depot M, Powell JR, Messenheimer JA Jr, et al. Kinetic effects of multiple oral doses of acetaminophen on a single oral dose of lamotrigine. Clin Pharmacol Ther 1990; 48:346–355.

14. Wong DD, Longenecker RG, Liepman M, et al. Phenytoin-dexamethasone: a possible drug-drug interaction. JAMA 1985; 254:2062–2063.

15. deAbajo FJ, Garcia-Rodriguez LA. Risk of upper gastrointestinal tract bleeding associated with selective serotonin reuptake inhibitors and venlafaxine therapy: interaction with nonsteroidal anti-inflammatory drugs and effect of acid-suppressing agents. Arch Gen Psychiatry 2008; 65:795–803.

16. Loke YK, Trivedi AN, Singh S. Meta-analysis: gastrointestinal bleeding due to interaction between selective serotonin reuptake inhibitors and non-steroidal anti-inflammatory drugs. Aliment Pharmacol Ther 2008; 27:31–40.

17. Graham DY, Malaty HM. Alendronate and naproxen are synergistic for development of gastric ulcers. Arch Intern Med 2001; 161:107–110.

18. Etminan M, Levesque L, Fitzgerald JM, Brophy JM. Risk of upper gastrointestinal bleeding with oral bisphosphonates and non steroidal anti-inflammatory drugs: a case-control study. Aliment Pharmacol Ther 2009; 29:1188–1192.

19. Pilgrim JL, Gerostamoulos D, Drummer OH. Deaths involving serotonergic drugs. Forensic Sci Int 2010; 198:110–117.

20. Mittino D, Mula M, Monaco F. Serotonin syndrome associated with tramadol-sertraline combination. Clin Neuropharmacol 2004; 27:150–151.

21. Houlihan DJ. Serotonin syndrome resulting from coadministration of tramadol, venlafaxine, and mirtazapine. Ann Pharmacother 2004; 38:411–413.

22. Gnanadesigan N, Espinoza RT, Smith R, et al. Interaction of serotonergic antidepressants and opioid analgesics: is serotonin syndrome going undetected? J Am Med Dir Assoc 2005; 6:265–269.

23. Ripple MG, Pestaner JP, Levine BS, Smialek JE. Lethal combination of tramadol and multiple drugs affecting serotonin. Am J Forensic Med Pathol 2000; 21:370–374.

24. Anonymous. Tapentadol (Nucynta) prescribing information. Raritan, NJ; Ortho-McNeil Janssen; July 2011.

25. Begre S, von Bardeleben U, Ladewig D, et al. Paroxetine increases steady-state concentrations of (r)—methadone in cyp2d6 extensive but not poor metabolizers. J Clin Psychopharmacol 2002; 22:211–215.

26. Iribarne C, Dreano Y, Bardou LG, et al. Interaction of methadone with substrates of human hepatic cytochrome p450 3a4. Toxicology 1997; 117:13–23.

27. Laugesen S, Enggaard TP, Pedersen RS, et al. Paroxetine, a cytochrome P450 2D6 inhibitor, diminishes the stereoselective O-demethylation and reduces the hypoalgesic effect of tramadol. Clin Pharmacol Ther 2005; 77:312–323.

28. Pilgrim JL, Gerostamoulos D, Drummer OH. Review: pharmacogenetic aspects of the effect of cytochrome P450 polymorphisms on serotonergic drug metabolism, response, interactions, and adverse effects. Forensic Sci Med Pathol 2011; 7:162–184.

29. Gwilt PR, Lear CL, Tempero MA, et al. The effect of garlic extract on human metabolism of acetaminophen. Cancer Epidemiol Biomarkers Prev 1994; 3:155–160.

30. Borrelli F, Capasso R, Izzo AA. Garlic (*Allium sativum* L.): adverse effects and drug interactions in humans. Mol Nutr Food Res 2007; 51:1386–1397.

31. Gardner CD, Zehnder JL, Rigby AJ, et al. Effect of Ginkgo biloba (EGb 761) and aspirin on platelet aggregation and platelet function among older adults at risk for cardiovascular disease: a randomized clinical trial. Blood Coagul Fibrinolysis 2007; 18:787–793.

32. Meisel C, Johne A, Roots I. Fatal intracerebral mass bleeding associated with Ginkgo biloba and ibuprofen. Atherosclerosis 2003; 167:367.

33. Kupiec T, Raj V. Fatal seizures due to potential herb-drug interactions with Ginkgo biloba. J Anal Toxicol 2005; 29:755–758.

34. Johne A, Schmider J, Brockmoller J, et al. Decreased plasma levels of amitriptyline and its metabolites on comedication with an extract from St. John's wort (*Hypericum perforatum*). J Clin Psychopharmacol 2002; 22:46–54.

35. Prost N, Tichadou L, Rodor F. et al. St. Johns wort-venlafaxine interaction. Presse Med 2000; 29:1285–1286.

36. Eich-Hochli D, Oppliger R, Golay KP, et al. Methadone maintenance treatment and St. John's wort: a case report. Pharmacopsychiatry 2003; 36:35–37.

Index

Note: Page numbers followed by f and t indicate figures and tables, respectively.

A

Acetaminophen, 9t
  adverse effects and side effects of, 3
  dosage and administration of, 3, 121
  garlic and, interactions between, 142t
  indications for, 3, 6, 6t, 8t
  intravenous, 121
  lamotrigine and, drug-drug interactions, 136t
  liver toxicity of, 3
  in multimodal analgesia, 121
  and opioids, combination therapy with, 121
  for postoperative pain, 121
    dosage and administration of, 127t
Acute pain service, 120
Adjuvant analgesic(s)
  for bone pain, 7, 7t
  for bowel obstruction, 7, 7t
  classification of, by clinical efficacy, 7, 7t
  definition of, 5
  multipurpose, 7, 7t
  for musculoskeletal pain, 7, 7t
  for neuropathic pain, 7, 7t
  and other analgesics, drug-drug interactions, 135t–138t
  on WHO analgesic/pain ladder, 2, 2f, 6, 6t
Adjuvant drug(s), definition of, 5
Adjuvant medicine(s), definition of, 5
α_2-Adrenergic agonists, 7t
  adverse effects and side effects of, 100
  for cancer pain, 96t, 99–100
  dosage and administration of, 99t
  mechanism of action of, 10t
α_1-Adrenergic receptor(s), as drug targets, 9t
α_2-Adrenergic receptor(s), as drug targets, 9t
Allergic reaction(s), 16, 18
  to local anesthetic, 55
  to methylparabene, 55
Allodynia, 11, 79
  definition of, 59–60
  intraoperative opioids and, 60–61
Amantadine
  for cancer pain, 96t
  for cancer-related neuropathic pain, 102
  mechanism of action of, 63
American Society of Anesthesiologists, guidelines for acute pain management in perioperative setting, 119, 126
Amitriptyline, 11
  adverse effects and side effects of, 12t, 81t
  for arthritis pain, 16
  for cancer pain, 88, 96t, 97–98
  dosage and administration of, 12t, 18, 80, 81t
  efficacy of, 14
  for fibromyalgia, 15, 17, 110
  half-life of, 12t
  for headache, 15–17
  for low back pain, 16
  mechanism of action of, 81t
  for neuropathic pain, 14, 17, 80, 81t, 88
  placebo-controlled trials of, 13t
  neurotransmitter profile of, 12t
  for postmastectomy pain, 88
  precautions with, 81t
  St. John's wort and, interactions between, 142t
  and serotonergic activity, 139t
  and sertraline, drug-drug interactions, 132t
  topical, 112
  venlafaxine and, drug-drug interactions, 141
Amphetamines, and serotonergic activity, 139t–140t
Analgesic(s)
  classification of
    by clinical efficacy, 5, 6t, 7, 7t
    mechanistic approaches for, 5, 6t, 7–8, 8t–9t
    by pain severity, 5–6, 6t
    by therapeutic class, 5, 6t, 7
  mechanistic taxonomy of, 8, 9t–10t
  multipurpose, for cancer pain, 95–96, 96t, 97–100, 99t
  serotonergic, 131–141, 139t
  topical. See Topical analgesics
Anandamide, 35f
Ankylosing spondylitis, pain of, treatment of, 16
Anorexia, AIDS-related, cannabinoids for, 34t
Antiarrhythmics, 7
  drug interactions with, 18
Antibiotic(s), drug interactions with, 18
Anticholinergics, 7t
  for cancer pain, 97t
  dosage and administration of, 99t

147

Anticholinergics (Cont.)
for cancer-related bowel obstruction, 103
Anticonvulsant(s), 5–7. See also specific drug
analgesic efficacy of, 21
for cancer pain, 96t
for fibromyalgia, 108–110, 109t
indications for, 8t
mechanism of action of, 21
for neuropathic pain, 86
cancer-related, 101
for rheumatic pain, 109t
Antidepressant(s), 5–7, 7t. See also specific drug
adverse effects and side effects of, 12t, 16
analgesic effects of, mechanism of action of, 13–14
anti-inflammatory effects of, 110
baseline tests with, 18
for cancer pain, 96t, 97–98, 99t
for chronic noncancer pain randomized controlled trials of, 11–17
selection of, 16–17
in combination therapy, 19
contraindications to, 17–18
dosage and administration of, 18–19
drug interactions with, 18
for fibromyalgia, 15, 108, 109t
for headache, 15–16
indications for, 8t
for low back pain, 16
mechanism of action of, 110
monitoring of therapy with, 18–19
for neuropathic pain, 14–15
cancer-related, 101
patient education about, 18
for postoperative pain, 124
dosage and administration of, 127t
precautions with, 111
for rheumatic pain, 109t, 110
serotonergic
and methadone, drug-drug interactions, 138t
and tapentadol, drug-drug interactions, 138t
and tramadol, drug-drug interactions, 138t
Antifungals, drug interactions with, 18
Antihyperalgesics, 9t
Antinociceptive analgesics, 9t
and modulators of descending inhibition/excitation, mixed, 10t
Anti-Parkinsonian drugs, 113
Antipsychotics, drug interactions with, 18
Antiretrovirals, drug interactions with, 18
Antispasmodics, indications for, 8t
Anxiety, improvement drugs for, 81t–82t
mirtazapine for, 98
Arrhythmia(s), local anesthetic-induced, 53–55
Arthritis pain, 11. See also Inflammatory arthritis; Osteoarthritis; Rheumatoid arthritis (RA)
treatment of, 16–17
Atropine, for cancer pain, 97t

B

Baclofen, 7t
for cancer pain, 97t
for cancer-related neuropathic pain, 102
Bisphosphonates, 5–6, 7t
adverse effects and side effects of, 102–103
for cancer pain, 97t
for cancer-related bone pain, 102–103
mechanism of action of, 10t, 102
oral
and multivalent cations, drug-drug interactions, 143
and NSAIDs, drug-drug interactions, 137t, 143
precautions with, 102–103
Bone pain
adjuvant analgesics for, 7, 7t
cancer-related
analgesics used for, 97t
bisphosphonates for, 102–103
calcitonin for, 97t, 103
dosage and administration of, 99t
clodronate for, 102–103
corticosteroids for, 98–99
ibandronate for, 102–103
monoclonal antibody for, 102–103
osteoclast inhibitor for, 102–103
pamidronate for, 102–103
radiopharmaceuticals for, 97t, 103
samarium-153 for, 97t, 103
strontium-89 for, 97t, 103
treatment of, 102–103
zolendronate for, 102–103
treatment of, 7, 7t
Botulinum toxin type A
for neuropathic pain, 89
for rheumatic pain, 112
Bowel obstruction pain
analgesics used for, 97t
dosage and administration of, 99t
cancer-related
analgesics used for, 97t
corticosteroids for, 98–99
treatment of, 103–104
treatment of, 7, 7t
Bupivacaine, 52
analgesic potency of, 52t
duration of action, 52t
maximum daily dose of, 55t
molecular structure of, 50–51, 51f
onset of action, 52t
pharmacology of, 50, 52t, 54f
for postoperative pain, dosage and administration of, 127t

Bupropion
  for cancer pain, 96t, 98
  contraindications to, 16
  for neuropathic pain, 14
Bursa block, 48t

C

Calcitonin, 7t
  for cancer-related bone pain, 97t, 103
  dosage and administration of, 99t
  mechanism of action of, 10t
Calcium channel $\alpha_2\delta$ ligands
  adverse effects and side effects of, 82t
  dosage and administration of, 82t, 84
  mechanism of action of, 82t, 84
  for neuropathic pain, 82t, 84
  precautions with, 82t
Calcium-channel blockers, drug interactions with, 18
Calcium channels, N-type, as drug targets, 9t
Camphor, 76
Cancer pain
  adjuvant analgesics used for, 95–96, 96t–97t
  α_2-adrenergic agonists for, 96t, 99–100
  dosage and administration of, 99t
  amantadine for, 96t
  amitriptyline for, 88, 96t, 97–98
  anticholinergics for, 97t
  dosage and administration of, 99t
  anticonvulsants for, 96t
  antidepressants for, 96t, 97–98, 99t
  atropine for, 97t
  baclofen for, 97t
  bisphosphonates for, 97t
  bupropion for, 96t, 98
  cannabinoids for, 34t, 39, 96t, 100
  dosage and administration of, 100
  carbamazepine for, 96t
  citalopram for, 96t
  clonazepam for, 97t
  clonidine for, 96t, 99–100
  corticosteroids for, 96t–97t, 98–99
  dosage and administration of, 99, 99t
  desipramine for, 96t, 97–98
  desvenlafaxine for, 96t
  dexamethasone for, 96t, 98–99
  dosage and administration of, 99, 99t
  dextromethorphan for, 96t
  divalproex for, 96t
  dronabinol for, 39, 96t, 100
  duloxetine for, 96t
  GABA agonists for, 97t
  gabapentin for, 96t
  glycopyrrolate for, 97t
  dosage and administration of, 99t
  ibandronate for, 97t
  intravenous lidocaine for, 96t
  ketamine for, 65, 96t
  lacosamide for, 96t
  lamotrigine for, 96t
  local anesthetics for, 96t
  memantine for, 96t
  methylprednisolone for, 98–99
  methylprednisone for, 96t
  mexiletine for, 96t
  milnacipran for, 96t
  multipurpose analgesics for, 95–96, 96t, 97–100, 99t
  nabilone for, 96t, 100
  nabiximols for, 96t, 100
  neuropathic. See Neuropathic pain, cancer-related
  NMDA receptor blockers (antagonists) for, 96t
  nortriptyline for, 96t
  NSAIDs for, 97t
  octreotide for, 97t
  dosage and administration of, 99t
  opioids for, 95
  osteoclast inhibitors for, 97t
  dosage and administration of, 99t
  oxcarbazepine for, 96t
  pamidronate for, 97t
  dosage and administration of, 99t
  paroxetine for, 96t
  phenytoin for, 96t
  prednisone for, 96t, 98–99
  dosage and administration of, 99, 99t
  pregabalin for, 96t
  prevalence of, 95
  scopolamine for, 97t
  SNRIs for, 96t, 97–98
  sodium channel blockers for, 96t
  sodium channel modulators for, 96t
  somatostatin analog for, 97t
  dosage and administration of, 99t
  SSRIs for, 96t
  tizanidine for, 96t, 99–100
  dosage and administration of, 99t
  topical analgesics for, 96t, 100
  topical capsaicin for, 96t, 100
  topical NSAIDs for, 96t
  topical tricyclic antidepressants for, 96t
  topiramate for, 96t
  treatment of, 2–3, 2f, 95
  tricyclic antidepressants for, 96t, 97–98
  undertreatment of, 95
  venlafaxine for, 96t, 98
  zolendronate for, 97t
Cancer treatment, local anesthetics and, 49
Cannabichromene, 33
Cannabidiol, 33. See also Cannabinoids
Cannabigerol, 33
Cannabinoid receptor, 33–36, 35f
Cannabinoids, 7t, 9t
  for acute pain, 36
  as adjuvant analgesics, 40–42
  adverse effects and side effects of, 39–40, 41t, 90, 111
  for AIDS-related anorexia, 34t

Cannabinoids *(Cont.)*
  analgesic efficacy of, 40–42
  antispasmodic effects of, 37–38
  anxiolytic effects of, 37
  available for medical practice, 33, 34t
  for cancer pain, 34t, 39, 96t, 100
    dosage and administration of, 100
  for chronic pain, 34t, 36–39
  dependence, 40, 41t, 90
  for fibromyalgia, 38–39, 109t, 111
  for HIV-related neuropathy, 36–37
  indications for, 8t
  mechanism of action of, 111
  for multiple sclerosis, 34t, 37–38
  for musculoskeletal pain, 38, 111
  for nausea and vomiting, in cancer chemotherapy, 34t
  for neuropathic pain, 15, 34t, 36–37
  and opioids
    combination therapy with, 40
    interactions of, 40
  oromucosal, for neuropathic pain, 89–90
  precautions with, 90
  for rheumatic pain, 109t
  for rheumatoid arthritis, 38, 111
  and sleep quality, 37–38
  for spinal cord injury, 37
Cannabinoid system, 33–36, 35f
Cannabinol, 33
Cannabis. *See* Marihuana (marijuana, cannabis)
Capsaicin
  mechanism of action of, 10t, 75, 83t, 85, 112
  molecular target of, 9t
  patch, 75
    adverse effects and side effects of, 83t
    dosage and administration of, 83t
    for HIV-related neuropathy, 83t, 88
    for neuropathic pain, 71, 83t, 85–86
  topical, 75–76
    adverse effects and side effects of, 75–76, 86
    for cancer pain, 96t, 100
    in combination therapy, 76
    for HIV-related neuropathy, 75–76, 85–86
    for rheumatic pain, 109t, 112
Carbamazepine, 23, 86
  adverse effects and side effects of, 23, 24t
  analgesic efficacy of, 21
  for cancer pain, 96t
  and codeine, drug-drug interactions, 136t
  contraindications to, 24t
  dosage and administration of, 24t
  and lamotrigine, drug-drug interactions, 133t
  mechanism of action of, 10t, 24t
  and methadone, drug-drug interactions, 135t
  molecular target of, 9t
  and phenytoin, drug-drug interactions, 133t
  precautions with, 24t
  and serotonergic activity, 139t
  and TCAs, drug-drug interactions, 133t
  for trigeminal neuralgia, 23, 86
  and valproate, drug-drug interactions, 132t
Cardiac arrest, local anesthetic-induced, 53–55
Catastrophizing, and neuropathic pain, 90
Cauda equina syndrome, local anesthetic-induced, 53–55
Causalgia, 8t
Celecoxib, for postoperative pain, dosage and administration of, 127t
Central sensitization, 8, 9t, 119
  evaluation of, 59–60
  intraoperative opioids and, 60–61
Cesamet. *See* Nabilone
Chemotherapy
  nausea and vomiting related to, cannabinoids for, 34t
  neuropathy caused by
    gabapentin for, 101
    management of, 80, 98
    pregabalin for, 101
Chloroprocaine
  analgesic potency of, 52t
  duration of action, 52t
  onset of action, 52t
  pharmacology of, 50, 52t
Chondroitin sulfate, 113
Cisapride, drug interactions with, 18
Cisplatin neuropathy, 14–15
Citalopram
  anti-inflammatory effects of, 110
  for cancer pain, 96t
  for fibromyalgia, 15
  for neuropathic pain, 14
  and serotonergic activity, 139t
  and serotonin syndrome, 141
Clodronate, for cancer-related bone pain, 102–103
Clomipramine
  adverse effects and side effects of, 12t
  dosage and administration of, 12t
  and fluvoxamine, drug-drug interactions, 132t
  half-life of, 12t
  and methadone, drug-drug interactions, 138t
  for neuropathic pain, placebo-controlled trials of, 13t
  neurotransmitter profile of, 12t
  and serotonergic activity, 139t
  and tapentadol, drug-drug interactions, 138t
  and tramadol, drug-drug interactions, 138t
Clonazepam, 28
  for cancer pain, 97t

for cancer-related
neuropathic pain,
102
Clonidine
adverse effects and side
effects of, 100
for cancer pain, 96t,
99–100
molecular target of, 9t
Coanalgesics, 6
definition of, 5
Cocaine
maximum daily dose
of, 55t
pharmacology of, 50
and serotonergic activity,
139t–140t
Codeine, 6, 6t
carbamazepine and,
drug-drug
interactions, 136t
Coeliac block, 2
Cognitive-behavioral
therapy, 1
Complementary and
alternative
medicine (CAM)
and analgesics,
interactions
between,
141–143, 142t
for rheumatic disease, 113
Complex regional pain
syndrome,
treatment of, 22
Constipation, drugs causing,
12t, 18
Corticosteroid(s), 7t
adverse effects and side
effects of, 98
for cancer pain, 96t–97t,
98–99
dosage and
administration of,
99, 99t
intra-articular injections,
112
intralesional injections,
112
joint injections, 112
local injection, for
rheumatic pain,
112
and opioids, combination
therapy with, 98
and phenytoin,
drug-drug
interactions, 136t
soft-tissue injections, 112
Counterirritants
mechanism of action of,
112
for rheumatic pain, 112

Coxibs, 9t, 121–122.
See also
Cyclooxygenase-2
(COX2) inhibitors
Cyclooxygenase-2 (COX2)
inhibitors, 9t
adverse effects and
side effects of,
121–122
contraindications to, 122
indications for, 3
for postoperative pain,
121–122
Cymbalta. See Duloxetine
Cystitis, 8t
Cytochrome P450
CYP2C19, anticonvulsants
metabolized by,
interactions with
gingko, 142t
CYP2D6
inhibitors
and TCAs, drug-drug
interactions, 134t
and tramadol,
drug-drug
interactions, 138t,
143
and tramadol
metabolism, 141
and venlafaxine
metabolism, 141
and drug-drug
interactions, 141,
143

D

Denosumab, for prevention
of skeletal
complications in
prostate cancer,
103
Depression
drugs for, 81t. See also
Antidepressant(s)
mirtazapine for, 98
Desipramine, 11
adverse effects and side
effects of, 12t, 81t
for cancer pain, 96t,
97–98
dosage and administration
of, 12t, 81t
efficacy of, 14
and fluvoxamine,
drug-drug
interactions, 132t
half-life of, 12t
mechanism of action
of, 81t
for neuropathic pain,
14, 81t

placebo-controlled
trials of, 13t
neurotransmitter profile
of, 12t
precautions with, 81t
and serotonergic activity,
139t
Desvenlafaxine, for cancer
pain, 96t
Dexamethasone
for cancer pain, 96t,
98–99
dosage and
administration of,
99, 99t
for pain emergencies, 99
Dextromethorphan, 63
for cancer pain, 96t
for cancer-related
neuropathic pain,
102
molecular target of, 9t
and serotonergic activity,
139t
Diabetic neuropathy, painful,
14–15, 17, 79–86
combination therapy
for, 89
duloxetine for, 81t
gabapentin for, 22, 82t
opioid agonists for, 83t,
85
pregabalin for, 22, 82t
topical capsaicin for,
75–76
topical lidocaine for, 74
tramadol for, 83t, 84
treatment of, 22–23, 27,
86, 88–89
tricyclic antidepressants
for, 81t
venlafaxine for, 81t
Diarrhea, drugs causing, 12t
Diclofenac
mechanism of action of, 72
patch, 72
topical
adverse effects and side
effects of, 72–73
gel, 72
randomized
controlled trials
of, 72–74, 73t
solution, with DMSO,
72
randomized
controlled trials
of, 72–74, 73t
Dietary therapy, for
rheumatic pain,
113
Divalproex. See also Sodium
divalproex

Divalproex *(Cont.)*
  for cancer pain, 96t
Dolasetron, for fibromyalgia, 113
Dopaminergic agents, 113
Douleur Neuropathique en 4 questions (DN4), 79
Doxepin
  adverse effects and side effects of, 12t
  dosage and administration of, 12t
  half-life of, 12t
  for low back pain, 16
  neurotransmitter profile of, 12t
  and serotonergic activity, 139t
Dronabinol, 36
  for cancer pain, 39, 96t, 100
  for chronic pain, 40
  dosage and administration of, 34t
  for fibromyalgia, 38
  indications for, 34t
  for MS-associated pain, 38
Drowsiness, drugs causing, 18
Drug-drug interactions. *See also specific drug*
  between adjuvant analgesics, 131, 132t–134t
  and other analgesics, 135t–138t
  with antidepressants, 18
  between herbals and analgesics, 141–143, 142t
  pharmacogenetics of, 131
  severity of, factors affecting, 131
Dry mouth, drugs causing, 12t, 18
Duloxetine, 5, 11
  adverse effects and side effects of, 12t, 81t
  for cancer pain, 96t
  for central neuropathic pain, 88
  dosage and administration of, 12t, 80, 81t, 110
  for fibromyalgia, 15, 17, 107, 109t
  half-life of, 12t
  for low back pain, 107, 110
  mechanism of action of, 81t
  for neuropathic pain, 14, 17, 80–84, 81t, 86

neurotransmitter profile of, 12t
and NSAIDs, drug-drug interactions, 137t, 143
for osteoarthritis pain, 107
and other serotonergic agents, drug-drug interactions, 143
for oxaliplatin-induced peripheral neuropathy, 98
for postoperative pain, dosage and administration of, 127t
precautions with, 81t
and serotonergic activity, 139t
and serotonin syndrome, 140

E

Ecstasy (drug)
  and serotonergic activity, 139t
  and serotonin syndrome, 141
Ectopic discharge, 8, 9t
Effexor. *See* Venlafaxine
Endocannabinoid system, 33–36, 35f
Epidural block, 3, 124, 125t
  and patient-controlled analgesia, comparison of, 124, 125t
Escitalopram, for neuropathic pain, 14
Etidocaine
  analgesic potency of, 52t
  duration of action, 52t
  onset of action, 52t
  pharmacology of, 52t
Eucalyptol, 76
European Society of Regional Anaesthesia, 126
Excitation, descending, modulators of, 9t
Exercise, in pan management, 1

F

Facial pain, 14
Failed back syndrome, 88
Felbamate, 28
Femoral nerve block, 48–49
Fenfluramine, and serotonergic activity, 139t

Fentanyl
  indications for, 6, 6t
  intranasal administration of, 122
  and other serotonergic agents, drug-drug interactions, 143
  in patient-controlled analgesia, 122
  and serotonergic activity, 139t
Fibromyalgia, 8t, 11, 14
  amitriptyline for, 15, 17, 110
  anticonvulsants for, 108–110, 109t
  antidepressants for, 15, 108, 109t
  cannabinoids for, 38–39, 109t, 111
  citalopram for, 15
  dolasetron for, 113
  dronabinol for, 38
  duloxetine for, 15, 17, 107, 109t
  fluoxetine for, 15
  gabapentin for, 22, 108–110, 109t
  gabapentinoids for, 108–110
  milnacipran for, 15, 17, 107, 109t
  moclobemide for, 15, 17
  monoamine oxidase inhibitors (MAOIs) for, 15, 17
  nabilone for, 38, 109t, 111
  nortriptyline for, 110
  paroxetine for, 15
  pathophysiology of, 107–108
  pirindole for, 15, 17
  pramipexole for, 113
  pregabalin for, 22–23, 107–110, 109t
  SNRIs for, 15, 17, 109t, 110
  SSRIs for, 15, 17, 109t
  treatment of, 15, 17, 21–23, 27, 107
  tricyclic antidepressants for, 17, 109t, 110
Flecainide, 49
Fluoxetine
  anti-inflammatory effects of, 110
  for fibromyalgia, 15
  and serotonergic activity, 139t
  and serotonin syndrome, 140–141

Fluvoxamine
  clomipramine and, drug-drug interactions, 132t
  desipramine and, drug-drug interactions, 132t
  imipramine and, drug-drug interactions, 132t
  and serotonergic activity, 139t
  tricyclic antidepressants and, drug-drug interactions, 132t, 134t

G

Gabapentin, 21–23, 74
  adverse effects and side effects of, 23, 82t
  analgesic efficacy of, 21
  for cancer pain, 96t
  for chronic noncancer pain, 17
  for diabetic neuropathy, 22, 82t
  dosage and administration of, 21–22, 82t, 84
  perioperative, 124
  and EMLA cream, combination therapy with, for neuropathic pain, cancer-related, 101
  for fibromyalgia, 22, 108–110, 109t
  gastroretentive formulation of, 22
    adverse effects and side effects of, 24t
    contraindications to, 24t
    dosage and administration of, 22, 24t
    mechanism of action of, 24t
    for postherpetic neuralgia, 22
    precautions with, 24t
  and imipramine, combination therapy with, for cancer-related neuropathic pain, 101
  immediate-release
    adverse effects and side effects of, 24t
    contraindications to, 24t
    dosage and administration of, 24t
    mechanism of action of, 24t
    precautions with, 24t
  indications for, 22
  mechanism of action of, 21, 82t, 84
  molecular target of, 9t
  and morphine, combination therapy with, for neuropathic pain, 89
  for neuropathic pain, 15, 17, 22–23, 82t, 84, 86, 88–89
    cancer-related, 101
    in hemodialysis patients, 23
  and nortriptyline, combination therapy with, for neuropathic pain, 88–89
  and opioids, combination therapy with, for cancer-related neuropathic pain, 101
  and oxycodone, combination therapy with, for neuropathic pain, 89
  pharmacology of, 21–22
  for postherpetic neuralgia, 22, 82t
  for postoperative pain, 123–124
    dosage and administration of, 127t
  precautions with, 82t
  for spinal cord injury-related pain, 82t, 86–88

Gabapentin enacarbil, 22
  adverse effects and side effects of, 24t
  contraindications to, 24t
  dosage and administration of, 22, 24t
  mechanism of action of, 24t
  precautions with, 24t

Gabapentinoids, 5, 7t, 9t, 13, 21–23
  adverse effects and side effects of, 110
  analgesic efficacy of, 21
  for chronic noncancer pain, 17
  for fibromyalgia, 108–110
  for neuropathic pain, 15, 17
    cancer-related, 101
  perioperative use of, 23
  for postoperative pain, 123–124
    dosage and administration of, 127t

Gamma-aminobutyric acid (GABA), as drug target, 9t
  in cancer-related neuropathic pain, 102

Gamma-aminobutyric acid (GABA) agonists, for cancer pain, 97t

Gamma knife ablation, 2

Garlic
  and acetaminophen, interactions between, 142t
  and NSAIDs, interactions between, 142t

Gastrointestinal distress, drugs causing, 12t

Gingko
  and anticonvulsants, interactions between, 142t
  and aspirin, interactions between, 142t
  and ibuprofen, interactions between, 142t

Glucosamine, 113

Glycopyrrolate
  for cancer pain, 97t
    dosage and administration of, 99t
  for cancer-related bowel obstruction, 103

Guanethidine block, molecular target of, 9t

Guarded receptor hypothesis, for local anesthetic action, 53, 54f

Guillain-Barré syndrome, 88

H

Headache, 11
  cancer-related, corticosteroids for, 98–99
  treatment of, 15–17

Hemodialysis patient(s), peripheral neuropathy in, treatment of, 23
Herbal therapy and analgesics, interactions between, 141–143, 142t
for rheumatic pain, 113
Herpes zoster, acute, treatment of, 22
Human immunodeficiency virus (HIV) neuropathy, 14–15
cannabinoids for, 36–37
capsaicin patch for, 83t
topical capsaicin for, 75–76, 85–86
treatment of, 22, 27, 88
Hyaluronic acid, intra-articular injections, for osteoarthritis in knee, 112–113
Hydrocodone, indications for, 6, 6t
Hydromorphone indications for, 6, 6t
in patient-controlled analgesia, 122
5-Hydroxytryptophan, and serotonergic activity, 139t
5-Hydroxytryptophan-1 receptor antagonists, and serotonergic activity, 139t
5-Hydroxytryptophan-3 receptor antagonists, 113
Hyperalgesia, 79
definition of, 59–60
intraoperative opioids and, 60–61
opioid-induced, 60–61, 61f, 85, 122–123
postoperative, 60
prevention, ketamine and, 123
primary, 59
secondary, 119
Hyponatremia, oxcarbazepine-induced, 25t

I

Ibandronate
for cancer pain, 97t
for cancer-related bone pain, 102–103

ID Pain, 79
Imipramine
adverse effects and side effects of, 12t
for arthritis pain, 16
and aspirin, drug-drug interactions, 135t
dosage and administration of, 12t
and fluvoxamine, drug-drug interactions, 132t
half-life of, 12t
and methadone, drug-drug interactions, 138t
for neuropathic pain, 14, 88
placebo-controlled trials of, 13t
neurotransmitter profile of, 12t
and phenytoin, drug-drug interactions, 132t
and serotonergic activity, 139t
and tapentadol, drug-drug interactions, 138t
and tramadol, drug-drug interactions, 138t
Incision block, 48t
Increased transmission mechanism, 8, 9t
Inflammatory arthritis pain of, mechanisms of, 107
pathophysiology of, 107–108
Inflammatory pain, 8t
cannabinoids for, 36
topical analgesics for, 71
Inhibition, descending, modulators of, 9t
Intercostal nerve block, 49
Intra-articular block, 2, 48t
Intrathecal analgesia, 2
Irritable bowel, 8t
pain from, treatment of, 22

J

Joint replacement, 2

K

Keratinocytes, as drug target, 76–77
Ketamine, 6
adverse effects and side effects of, 63
anti-hyperalgesic effect of, 61–63

for cancer pain, 65, 96t
for cancer-related neuropathic pain, 101–102
benzodiazepine with, 102
dosage and administration of, 101–102
neuroleptic with, 102
for chronic pain, 64–65
dosage and administration of, 64–65, 123
effects on postoperative opioid consumption, 61–62
effects on postoperative pain, 61–63
epidural, 62
intravenous, dosage and administration of, recommendations for, 62, 62t
mechanism of action of, 61, 123
molecular target of, 9t
for opioid-induced hyperalgesia, 122–123
and opioids, in same solution for PCA, 63
perioperative benefits of, 61–63
dosage and administration of, recommendations for, 62, 62t
indications for, 63
pharmacology of, 61, 64–65
for postoperative pain, 123
dosage and administration of, 127t
for rheumatic pain, 112
S(+), 62

L

Lacosamide, 27–28, 86
adverse effects and side effects of, 26t
for cancer pain, 96t
for cancer-related neuropathic pain, 101
dosage and administration of, 26t
mechanism of action of, 26t

Laminectomy, 2
Lamotrigine, 9t, 27
  and acetaminophen, drug-drug interactions, 136t
  adverse effects and side effects of, 25t
  for cancer pain, 96t
  for cancer-related neuropathic pain, 101
  carbamazepine and, drug-drug interactions, 133t
  contraindications to, 25t
  dosage and administration of, 25t
  for HIV-related neuropathy, 88
  mechanism of action of, 25t
  molecular target of, 9t
  for neuropathic pain, 88
  and phenytoin, drug-drug interactions, 134t
  precautions with, 25t
Leeds Assessment of Neuropathic Symptoms and Signs (LANSS), 79
Leukopenia, drugs causing, 23
Levetiracetam, 9t, 27
  adverse effects and side effects of, 26t
  dosage and administration of, 26t
  mechanism of action of, 26t
Levobupivacaine
  analgesic potency of, 52t
  duration of action, 52t
  maximum daily dose of, 55t
  onset of action, 52t
  pharmacology of, 52t
  for postoperative pain, dosage and administration of, 127t
Levorphanol
  adverse effects and side effects of, 83t
  dosage and administration of, 83t
  mechanism of action of, 83t
  for neuropathic pain, 83t, 88
  precautions with, 83t
Lidocaine
  analgesic potency of, 52t
  duration of action, 52t, 53
  intravenous, 49, 53
    for cancer pain, 96t
    for cancer-related neuropathic pain, 101
  maximum daily dose of, 55t
  mechanism of action of, 74, 82t
  molecular target of, 9t
  onset of action, 52t
  patch, 49, 74
  pharmacology of, 50, 52t, 54f
  plaster, 74
    for neuropathic pain, 84
  subcutaneous, for cancer-related neuropathic pain, 101
  topical, 74–75
    adverse effects and side effects of, 82t, 84
    dosage and administration of, 82t, 84
    indications for, 74–75
    and lidocaine gel, mixture of, 49–50
    for neuropathic pain, 82t, 84
    and oral therapy, combination of, 75
    pharmacology of, 74
    for postherpetic neuralgia, 74, 82t, 86
Lithium, and serotonergic activity, 139t
Local anesthetics, 6, 47. See also specific drug
  administration of
    routes for, 47, 48t
    systemic, 47, 49
    techniques for, 47, 48t
    topical, 47, 48t, 49–50
    ultrasound-guided, 47
  adverse effects and side effects of
    class A, 53
    class B, 53–55
  amino amide, 50
    pharmacology of, 52t
  amino ester, 50
    pharmacology of, 52t
  anesthetic potency of, 50–51
  anti-inflammatory action of, 49
  for cancer pain, 96t
  in cancer treatment, 49
  contraindications to, 50
  differential block of sensory and motor fibers, 51–52
  dosage and administration of, 51
  duration of action, 50–51
    and toxicological profile, 50, 53
  epidural analgesia with, for postoperative pain, 124, 125t
  eutectic mixture of, 49–50
  guarded receptor hypothesis for, 53, 54f
  hydrophobicity of, 50–51, 53, 54f
  inadvertent systemic application of, 53
  infusions, for postoperative pain, 124
  intra-articular infusion, for postoperative pain, 125
  liposomal formulations, 125
  maximum daily dose of, 55t
  mechanism of action of, 10t, 47–49
  octanol-buffer coefficient of, 53, 54f
  onset of action, 50–51
    and toxicological profile, 50, 53
  pharmacology of, 50–52, 52t
  for postoperative pain, dosage and administration of, 127t
  precautions with, 50
  safety of, 47
  toxicity of, 53–56
    clinical signs of, 55, 56t
    lipid rescue therapy for, 53, 55–56
    management protocols for, 56
  wound infiltration with, 124
Low back pain, 11
  treatment of, 16–17, 27, 107, 110
Lumbar radicular pain, treatment of, 27
Lumbar root pain, chronic, 14–15

Lumbar spinal stenosis, pain of, treatment of, 22
Lymphedema, cancer-related, corticosteroids for, 98–99

M

Macrolides, drug interactions with, 18
Magnesium
 as NMDA receptor blocker, 63–64
 and perioperative pain management, 63–64
Maprotiline, 11
 for neuropathic pain, 14
Marihuana (marijuana, cannabis), 34t. See also Cannabinoids
 medical use of, 33, 111
  vs. recreational use, 111
 smoked
  for HIV-related neuropathy, 37, 88
  for neuropathic pain, 36–37
 synthetic derivatives of, 33, 34t
Marinol. See Dronabinol
Massage, 1
MDMA
 and serotonergic activity, 139t
 and serotonin syndrome, 141
Memantine
 for cancer pain, 96t
 for cancer-related neuropathic pain, 102
 mechanism of action of, 63
Menthol, 76
 for rheumatic pain, 112
Meperidine
 and other serotonergic agents, drug-drug interactions, 143
 and serotonergic activity, 139t
Mepivacaine, 52–53
 analgesic potency of, 52t
 duration of action, 52t
 molecular structure of, 50–51, 51f
 onset of action, 52t
 pharmacology of, 50, 52t

Methadone
 adverse effects and side effects of, 83t
 carbamazepine and, drug-drug interactions, 135t
 clomipramine and, drug-drug interactions, 138t
 dosage and administration of, 83t
 drug interactions with, 18
 imipramine and, drug-drug interactions, 138t
 indications for, 6, 6t
 mechanism of action of, 63, 83t
 mirtazapine and, drug-drug interactions, 138t
 for neuropathic pain, 83t, 85
 and other serotonergic agents, drug-drug interactions, 138t, 143
 precautions with, 83t
 St. John's wort and, interactions between, 142t
 and serotonergic activity, 139t
 and serotonin syndrome, 140
 SSRIs and, drug-drug interactions, 138t
 trazodone and, drug-drug interactions, 138t
 venlafaxine and, drug-drug interactions, 138t, 141
N-Methyl-D-aspartate (NMDA) receptor(s)
 activation of, 60
 in opioid-induced hyperalgesia, 122
 and μ-opioid receptors, link between, 61, 61f
 and postoperative hyperalgesia, 60–61, 61f
N-Methyl-D-aspartate (NMDA) receptor blockers (antagonists), 7t, 9t, 14, 113
 for cancer pain, 96t
 for cancer-related neuropathic pain, 101–102

 for chronic pain, 64–65
 for neuropathic pain, 59
 for postoperative pain, 59
Methylparabene, allergic reactions to, 55
Methylprednisolone, for cancer pain, 98–99
Methylprednisone, for cancer pain, 96t
Mexiletine
 for cancer pain, 96t
 molecular target of, 9t
 oral, 49
Migraine, treatment of, 15–17
Milnacipran, 11
 for cancer pain, 96t
 for fibromyalgia, 15, 17, 107, 109t
Mind-body interventions, 1
Mindfulness, in pan management, 1
Mirtazapine
 for cancer-related symptoms, 98
 for headache, 15–17
 and methadone, drug-drug interactions, 138t
 and tapentadol, drug-drug interactions, 138t
 and tramadol, drug-drug interactions, 138t
Moclobemide
 for fibromyalgia, 15, 17
 and serotonergic activity, 139t
Monoamine oxidase inhibitors (MAOIs)
 for fibromyalgia, 15, 17
 and serotonergic activity, 139t
Monoclonal antibody(ies) (mAb), for cancer-related bone pain, 102–103
Morphine
 adverse effects and side effects of, 83t
 for chronic noncancer pain, 17
 dosage and administration of, 83t
 indications for, 6, 6t
 intrathecal, 124
 long-term administration, problems caused by, 85
 mechanism of action of, 83t

for neuropathic pain, 15, 83t, 85
in patient-controlled analgesia, 122
precautions with, 83t
Multimodal analgesia, 121
Multiple sclerosis (MS), pain in, 27
cannabinoids for, 34t, 37–38
treatment of, 22
Muscle relaxant(s), 5–7
Muscle spasm(s), in spinal cord injury, cannabinoids for, 37
Musculoskeletal pain, 8t. See also Fibromyalgia; Rheumatic pain
cannabinoids for, 38, 111
treatment of, 7, 7t

N

Nabilone, 36–37
adverse effects and side effects of, 111
for cancer pain, 96t, 100
dosage and administration of, 34t
for fibromyalgia, 38, 109t, 111
indications for, 34t
for musculoskeletal pain, 38
Nabiximols
adverse effects and side effects of, 34t
for cancer pain, 96t, 100
dosage and administration of, 34t
indications for, 34t
Naproxen, for postoperative pain, dosage and administration of, 127t
Nausea and vomiting
chemotherapy-related, cannabinoids for, 34t
drugs causing, 12t
postoperative, prevention, 123–124
Nefazodone, and serotonergic activity, 139t
Nefopam, 9t
Nerve block(s), 2–3, 47, 48t
adverse effects and side effects of, 55
differential, 52
for postoperative pain, 124–125, 125t

Neuralgia, 8t
Neuraxial block(s), 48, 48t, 124, 125t
Neurolytic block, 3
Neuropathic pain, 5, 8, 8t, 11
adjuvant analgesics for, 7, 7t
amitriptyline for, 14, 17, 80, 81t, 88
placebo-controlled trials of, 13t
anticonvulsants for, 86
antidepressants for, 14–15
botulinum toxin type A for, 89
bupropion for, 14
calcium channel $\alpha_2\delta$ ligands for, 82t, 84
cancer-related, 14. See also Cancer pain
amantadine for, 102
amitriptyline for, 88
analgesics used for, 96t–97t
anticonvulsants for, 101
antidepressants for, 101
baclofen for, 102
clonazepam for, 102
corticosteroids for, 98–99
dextromethorphan for, 102
gabapentin for, 82t, 101
gabapentin and EMLA cream for, combination therapy with, 101
gabapentin and imipramine for, combination therapy with, 101
gabapentin and opioids for, combination therapy with, 101
gabapentinoids for, 101
intravenous lidocaine for, 101
ketamine for, 101–102
benzodiazepine with, 102
dosage and administration of, 101–102
neuroleptic with, 102
lacosamide for, 101
lamotrigine for, 101
memantine for, 102
NMDA receptor blockers (antagonists) for, 101–102
oxcarbazepine for, 101

pregabalin for, 101
sodium channel blockers for, 101
sodium divalproex for, 101
subcutaneous lidocaine for, 101
topiramate for, 101
treatment of, 22, 100–102
tricyclic antidepressants for, 81t
in cancer survivors, 100–101
cannabinoids for, 15, 34t, 36–37, 89–90
oromucosal, 89–90
capsaicin patch for, 71, 83t, 85–86
catastrophizing and, 90
central, 86–88
duloxetine for, 88
characteristics of, 79
citalopram for, 14
clomipramine for, placebo-controlled trials of, 13t
combination therapy for, 75–76, 88–89
desipramine for, 14, 81t
placebo-controlled trials of, 13t
diagnosis of, 79–80
duloxetine for, 14, 17, 80–84, 81t, 86
escitalopram for, 14
etiology of, 79
evoked, 79, 90
gabapentin for, 15, 17, 22–23, 82t, 84, 86, 88–89
in hemodialysis patients, 23
and morphine, combination therapy with, 89
and nortriptyline, combination therapy with, 88–89
and oxycodone, combination therapy with, 89
gabapentinoids for, 15, 17
imipramine for, 14, 88
placebo-controlled trials of, 13t
intensity, temporal variations in, 79
intermittent, 79
lamotrigine for, 88
levorphanol for, 83t, 88

Neuropathic pain *(Cont.)*
lidocaine plaster for, 84
management of, 49
adjuvant analgesics for, 81t–83t
evidence-based recommendations for, 81t–83t
maprotiline for, 14
methadone for, 83t, 85
morphine for, 15, 83t, 85
NMDA receptor blockers (antagonists) for, 59
nortriptyline for, 14, 17, 81t, 88
placebo-controlled trials of, 13t
opioid agonists for, 83t, 85
opioids for, 15
oxycodone for, 15, 83t, 85
paroxetine for, 14
pathophysiologic heterogeneity of, 90
peripheral, 80–86
treatment algorithm for, 87f
pregabalin for, 15, 17, 22–23, 74–75, 82t, 84, 86, 88
and duloxetine, combination therapy with, 22, 89
in hemodialysis patients, 23
prevalence of, 79
psychological comorbidity and, 90
screening tools for, 79–80
smoked cannabis for, 36–37
SNRIs for, 14–15, 17, 80–84, 81t
spontaneous, 79
SSRIs for, 14–15
placebo-controlled trials of, 13t
tapentadol for, 85
tetracyclic antidepressant for, 14
therapeutic outcomes in, improving, 90
topical analgesics for, 71, 74–76
topical lidocaine for, 74–75, 82t, 84
tramadol for, 15, 83t, 84
traumatic, 79
treatment of, 88
tricyclic antidepressants for, 81t

treatment of, 7, 7t, 14–15, 17, 21, 27
clinical trials, factors affecting, 90
placebo-controlled trials of, 13t
placebo effect in, 90
tricyclic antidepressants for, 14–15, 17, 80, 81t, 88–89
placebo-controlled trials of, 13t
venlafaxine for, 14, 17, 80–84, 81t, 88
placebo-controlled trials of, 13t
Neuropathic Pain Questionnaire, 79
Nitrous oxide, 9t
anti-hyperalgesic effect of, 64
as NMDA receptor blocker, 64
Nociception, 48
Nociceptive pain, 8, 8t, 47–48
Nociceptor(s), 48
Nonopioid(s), 9t
indications for, 3
on WHO analgesic/pain ladder, 2, 2f, 6, 6t
Nonsteroidal anti-inflammatory drugs (NSAIDs), 9t. *See also specific drug*
adverse effects and side effects of, 3, 121–122
for cancer pain, 97t
contraindications to, 122
indications for, 3, 6, 6t, 8t
and morphine, combination therapy with, 121–122
in multimodal analgesia, 121–122
oral bisphosphonates and, drug-drug interactions, 137t, 143
for postoperative pain, 121–122
dosage and administration of, 127t
topical, 71–74, 73t. *See also* Diclofenac, topical
for cancer pain, 96t
mechanism of action of, 112

for rheumatic pain, 109t, 112
Norfluoxetine, and serotonin syndrome, 140–141
Nortriptyline, 11
adverse effects and side effects of, 12t, 81t
for cancer pain, 96t
dosage and administration of, 12t, 18, 81t
efficacy of, 14
for fibromyalgia, 110
half-life of, 12t
for low back pain, 16
mechanism of action of, 81t
for neuropathic pain, 14, 17, 81t, 88
placebo-controlled trials of, 13t
neurotransmitter profile of, 12t
precautions with, 81t

O

Octreotide, 7t
for cancer pain, 97t
dosage and administration of, 99t
for cancer-related bowel obstruction, 103–104
Ofirmev, 121
Opioid(s), 9t. *See also* Hyperalgesia, opioid-induced; *specific drug*
abuse, 4
adverse effects and side effects of, 122
and cannabinoids combination therapy with, 40
interactions of, 40
for chronic noncancer pain, 17
combinations of, efficacy of, 3
dependence, 85
diversion, 4
dosage and administration of, 3
indications for, 3–4, 8t
intraoperative, 60–61
long-term administration, problems caused by, 85
for neuropathic pain, 15
and NMDA receptor activation, 60

for phantom limb pain, 88
for postoperative pain, 122
response to, factors affecting, 3–4
rotation of, 4
serotonergic
and other serotonergic agents, drug-drug interactions, 143
and serotonin syndrome, 140
and serotonergic activity, 139t
spinal
adverse effects and side effects of, 124
for postoperative pain, 124
strong, on WHO analgesic/pain ladder, 2–3, 2f, 6, 6t
weak, on WHO analgesic/pain ladder, 2–3, 2f, 6, 6t
Opioid agonist(s)
adverse effects and side effects of, 83t, 85
dosage and administration of, 83t
mechanism of action of, 83t
for neuropathic pain, 83t, 85
precautions with, 83t, 85
μ-Opioid agonists, 9t
μ-Opioid receptor(s)
as drug targets, 9t
and NMDA receptors, link between, 61, 61f
Orthostatic hypotension, drugs causing, 12t
Osteoarthritis
in knee, intra-articular hyaluronic acid for, 112–113
pain of
herbal therapy for, 113
mechanisms of, 107
neurogenic mechanisms in, 108
pathophysiology of, 107–108
topical analgesics for, 112
topical capsaicin for, 75
topical diclofenac for, 72–74, 73t
treatment of, 16, 107

Osteoclast inhibitor(s). See also Bisphosphonates
for cancer pain, 97t
dosage and administration of, 99t
for cancer-related bone pain, 102–103
Oxcarbazepine, 23, 86
adverse effects and side effects of, 23, 25t
for cancer pain, 96t
for cancer-related neuropathic pain, 101
contraindications to, 25t
dosage and administration of, 25t
mechanism of action of, 10t, 25t
precautions with, 25t
Oxycodone
adverse effects and side effects of, 83t
for chronic noncancer pain, 17
dosage and administration of, 83t, 85
high-dose, indications for, 6, 6t
low-dose, indications for, 6, 6t
mechanism of action of, 83t
for neuropathic pain, 15, 83t, 85
precautions with, 83t

P

Pain
acute
management of, 2–3, 36
topical diclofenac for, 72
arthritis. See Arthritis pain
bone. See Bone pain
cancer. See Cancer pain
central poststroke, 14, 27, 79
tricyclic antidepressants for, 81t
chronic, 11
acute crises, management of, 3
cannabinoids for, 34t, 36–39
management of, 3, 34t, 36–40, 64–65
NMDA receptor modulators for, 64–65
postoperative, 126

without control, management of, 3
definition of, 1
mild, treatment of, 2, 2f, 3, 6, 6t
moderate, treatment of, 2, 2f, 3–4, 6, 6t
musculoskeletal. See Musculoskeletal pain
neuropathic. See Neuropathic pain
nonmalignant, management of, 2–3
postamputation, treatment of, 100
postmastectomy
gabapentin and EMLA cream combination therapy for, 101
treatment of, 88, 98, 100
postsurgical, 79. See also Postoperative pain
chronic, 126
treatment of, 23
postthoracotomy, treatment of, 22, 100
rheumatic. See Osteoarthritis; Rheumatic pain; Rheumatoid arthritis (RA)
severe, treatment of, 2, 2f, 3–4, 6, 6t
PainDetect, 79
Pain emergencies, 99
Pain management
approaches to
interventional, 1–2
invasive, 2–3
nonpharmacological, 1
pharmacological, 2–3
physical, 1
psychological, 1
specific, 2
step down, 3
step up, 3
for chronic pain, 3. See also Pain, chronic
step-down approach, 3
step-up approach, 3
goals of, 1
Pamidronate
for cancer pain, 97t
dosage and administration of, 99t
for cancer-related bone pain, 102–103

Pancreatitis, chronic, pain from, treatment of, 22
Paravertebral block, 48t
Parietal block(s), 48t
Paroxetine
 for cancer pain, 96t
 for fibromyalgia, 15
 for neuropathic pain, 14
 and serotonergic activity, 139t
 and serotonin syndrome, 141
 and tramadol, drug-drug interactions, 138t
Patient-controlled analgesia (PCA), 3
 and epidural analgesia, comparison of, 124, 125t
 for postoperative pain, 122
Penile nerve block (dorsal), 48t
Perfalgan, 121
Perineural analgesia, for postoperative pain, 124
Peripheral nerve(s), transmission of nociceptive information, 48–49
Peripheral nerve block, 2, 48, 48t, 124, 125t
Peripheral neuropathy
 chemotherapy-related, pregabalin for, 101
 local anesthetic-induced, 53–55
 oxaliplatin-induced, treatment of, 98
Peripheral sensitization, 8, 9t, 119
 evaluation of, 59–60
 modulators of, 10t
Peripheral transmission, modulators of, 10t
Phantom limb pain, 14
 opioid agonists for, 83t
 tramadol for, 83t
 treatment of, 88
Phenelzine, and serotonergic activity, 139t
Phentolamine, molecular target of, 9t
Phenytoin, 28
 for cancer pain, 96t
 carbamazepine and, drug-drug interactions, 133t
 corticosteroids and, drug-drug interactions, 136t
 imipramine and, drug-drug interactions, 132t
 lamotrigine and, drug-drug interactions, 134t
 tricyclic antidepressants and, drug-drug interactions, 132t
Pirindole, for fibromyalgia, 15, 17
Plexus block, 48t, 49, 124, 125t
Polyneuropathy, 14, 27
Postherpetic neuralgia, 14–15, 17, 79–86
 capsaicin patch for, 83t
 combination therapy for, 89
 gabapentin for, 22, 82t
 nerve block for, 49
 opioid agonists for, 83t, 85
 pregabalin for, 22, 82t
 topical capsaicin for, 75–76, 85–86
 topical lidocaine for, 74, 82t, 84
 treatment of, 22–23, 86, 88–89
 tricyclic antidepressants for, 81t
Postoperative pain
 acetaminophen for, 121
  dosage and administration of, 127t
 acute, 119
  management of, 120–126
  ASA guidelines for, 119
  multidisciplinary approach to (acute pain service), 120
 antidepressants for, 124
  dosage and administration of, 127t
 balanced analgesia for, 121
 bupivacaine for, dosage and administration of, 127t
 celecoxib for, dosage and administration of, 127t
 chronic, 119, 126
  prevalence of, 126
  risk factors for, 126
 COX2 inhibitors for, 121–122
 duloxetine for, dosage and administration of, 127t
 gabapentin for, 123–124
  dosage and administration of, 127t
 gabapentinoids for, 123–124
  dosage and administration of, 127t
 ketamine for, 61–63, 123
  dosage and administration of, 127t
  effects on opioid consumption, 61–62
 levobupivacaine for, dosage and administration of, 127t
 local anesthetics for, 124–125, 127t
 long-term, 60
 management of, 36, 120–126
 multimodal analgesia for, 121
 naproxen for, dosage and administration of, 127t
 nerve block for, 124–125, 125t
 NMDA receptor blockers (antagonists) for, 59
 nonopioid drugs for, dosage and administration of, 127t
 NSAIDs for, 121–122
  dosage and administration of, 127t
 opioids for, 122
  spinal, 124
 pathophysiology of, 119–120
 patient-controlled analgesia (PCA) for, 122
 perception of, factors affecting, 120t
 perineural analgesia for, 124
 pregabalin for, 123–124
  dosage and administration of, 127t
 procedure-specific guidelines for, 125–126

regional anesthesia for, 124–125, 125t
ropivacaine for, dosage and administration of, 127t
venlafaxine for, dosage and administration of, 127t
Posttraumatic pain. *See also* Neuropathic pain, traumatic
chronic, 119
Pramipexole
adverse effects and side effects of, 113
for fibromyalgia, 113
Prednisone
for cancer pain, 96t, 98–99
dosage and administration of, 99, 99t
and NSAIDs, drug-drug interactions, 137t
Pregabalin, 5, 9t, 21–23
adverse effects and side effects of, 23, 24t, 82t, 123
analgesic efficacy of, 21
for cancer pain, 96t
and celecoxib, combination therapy with
for back pain, 110
for postsurgical pain, 23
for chronic noncancer pain, 17
contraindications to, 24t
dosage and administration of, 21–23, 24t, 82t, 84
perioperative, 124
and duloxerine, combination therapy with, for neuropathic pain, 89
and duloxetine, combination therapy with, for chronic peripheral neuropathic pain, 22
for fibromyalgia, 22–23, 107–110, 109t
indications for, 22
mechanism of action of, 21, 24t, 82t, 84
for neuropathic pain, 15, 17, 22–23, 74–75, 82t, 84, 86, 88
cancer-related, 101

in hemodialysis patients, 23
for osteoarthritis pain, 110
for painful diabetic neuropathy, 22, 82t
perioperative use of, 123
pharmacology of, 21–22
for postherpetic neuralgia, 22, 82t
for postoperative pain, 123–124
dosage and administration of, 127t
for posttraumatic neuropathy, 88
precautions with, 24t, 82t
for spinal cord injury-related pain, 22, 86–88
Prilocaine, 52
analgesic potency of, 52t
duration of action, 52t
and lignocaine, mixture of, 49–50
maximum daily dose of, 55t
onset of action, 52t
pharmacology of, 50, 52t
Procaine
analgesic potency of, 52t
duration of action, 52t
onset of action, 52t
pharmacology of, 50, 52t
PROSPECT working group, 126
Prostate cancer, skeletal complications of, denosumab for, 103

Q

Quetenza. *See* Capsaicin, patch
Quinolones, drug interactions with, 18

R

Radial nerve block, 48
Radiculopathy, 8t, 79
chronic, treatment of, 88
lumbosacral, 88
transient, local anesthetic-induced, 53–55
Radiopharmaceuticals, 7t
for cancer-related bone pain, 97t, 103
RANKL, monoclonal antibodies that inhibit, 102–103

Rasagiline, and serotonergic activity, 139t
Reduced inhibition mechanism, 8, 9t
Referred pain, 119
Regional anesthesia, 47
adverse effects and side effects of, 55
intraoperative, 61
for postoperative pain, 124–125, 125t
Restless legs, 113
Rheumatic pain. *See also* Fibromyalgia; Musculoskeletal pain; Osteoarthritis; Rheumatoid arthritis (RA)
causes of, 107–108
neurogenic mechanisms in, 108
topical analgesics for, 112–113
Rheumatism, soft-tissue, 107–108
Rheumatoid arthritis (RA), pain of
cannabinoids for, 38, 111
topical capsaicin for, 75
treatment of, 16
Rib fracture(s), pain caused by, nerve block for, 49
Ropivacaine, 52
analgesic potency of, 52t
duration of action, 52t
maximum daily dose of, 55t
molecular structure of, 50–51, 51f
onset of action, 52t
pharmacology of, 50, 52t, 54f
for postoperative pain, dosage and administration of, 127t

S

St. John's wort
and amitriptyline, interactions between, 142t
and methadone, interactions between, 142t
and serotonergic activity, 139t–140t
and venlafaxine, interactions between, 142t

Samarium-153, for cancer-related bone pain, 97t, 103
Sativex. See also Nabiximols
 for rheumatic pain, 109t
 for rheumatoid arthritis, 111
Sciatic nerve block, 48–49
Scopolamine
 for cancer pain, 97t
 for cancer-related bowel obstruction, 103
Sedation, drugs causing, 12t, 16, 18
Seizure(s)
 nerve block and, 55
 tramadol and, 84
Selective serotonin reuptake inhibitors (SSRIs), 11, 14. See also specific drug
 for cancer pain, 96t
 for chronic noncancer pain, 17–19
 drug interactions with, 18
 for fibromyalgia, 15, 17, 109t
 for headache, 15–16
 mechanism of action of, 10t
 and methadone, drug-drug interactions, 138t
 for neuropathic pain, 14–15
 placebo-controlled trials of, 13t
 and NSAIDs, drug-drug interactions, 137t
 and serotonergic activity, 139t
 and serotonin syndrome, 140
 and tapentadol, drug-drug interactions, 138t
 and tramadol, drug-drug interactions, 138t
Selegiline, and serotonergic activity, 139t
Serotonergic activity, drugs enhancing, 131–141, 139t–140t
Serotonergic agents, two or more, combination therapy with, drug-drug interactions in, 143
Serotonin-norepinephrine reuptake inhibitors (SNRIs), 11–13, 12t, 14. See also specific drug

adverse effects and side effects of, 16
for cancer pain, 96t, 97–98
for chronic noncancer pain, 17–19
for fibromyalgia, 15, 17, 109t, 110
for headache, 15–16
mechanism of action of, 9t, 81t
for neuropathic pain, 14–15, 17, 80–84, 81t
precautions with, 81t
for rheumatic pain, 109t, 110
and serotonergic activity, 139t
and serotonin syndrome, 140
Serotonin syndrome, 84, 131–141, 138t, 143
 deaths from, 141
Serotonin toxicity, 131–141
Sertraline
 and serotonergic activity, 139t
 and serotonin syndrome, 141
Sexual dysfunction, drugs causing, 18
Shock-wave therapy, 1
Sleep disturbance
 calcium channel blockers and, 82t
 cannabinoids for, 37–38
 mirtazapine for, 98
 SNRIs for, 81t
Sodium channel
 tetrodotoxin-resistant-voltage gated, as drug target, 9t
 tetrodotoxin-sensitive-voltage gated, as drug target, 9t
Sodium channel blocker(s), 7t, 14
 for cancer pain, 96t
 for cancer-related neuropathic pain, 101
 indications for, 8t
 molecular target of, 9t
 oral, 49
Sodium channel modulator(s), for cancer pain, 96t
Sodium divalproex. See also Divalproex

Sodium divalproex, for cancer-related neuropathic pain, 101
Somatic pain, 8t
Somatostatin analog
 for cancer pain, 97t
 dosage and administration of, 99t
 for cancer-related bowel obstruction, 103–104
Spasticity
 in multiple sclerosis, cannabinoids for, 37–38
 in spinal cord injury, cannabinoids for, 37
Spinal block, 2, 124, 125t
 adverse effects and side effects of, 55
Spinal cord, transmission of nociceptive information by, 49
Spinal cord injury pain, 14–15, 79
 cannabinoids for, 37
 gabapentin for, 82t, 86–88
 management cannabinoids for, 37
 pregabalin for, 22, 82t, 86–88
 tramadol for, 83t, 86–88
 treatment of, 22, 86–88
 tricyclic antidepressants for, 81t, 86–88
Spinal stimulator, 3
Steroid(s), 5–6
 indications for, 8t
Stevens-Johnson syndrome, drugs causing, 23, 24t
Strontium-89, for cancer-related bone pain, 97t, 103
Subcostal nerve block, 49
Sumatriptan, and serotonergic activity, 139t
Sympathetically maintained pain, 8, 9t
Sympathetic nerve block, 2

T

Tamoxifen, drug interactions with, 18
Tapentadol
 clomipramine and, drug-drug interactions, 138t

dosage and administration of, 85
imipramine and, drug-drug interactions, 138t
mechanism of action of, 10t, 85
mirtazapine and, drug-drug interactions, 138t
for neuropathic pain, 85
and other serotonergic agents, drug-drug interactions, 138t, 143
and serotonergic activity, 139t
SSRIs and, drug-drug interactions, 138t
trazodone and, drug-drug interactions, 138t
venlafaxine and, drug-drug interactions, 138t

Tetracaine
analgesic potency of, 52t
duration of action, 52t
onset of action, 52t
pharmacology of, 50, 52t

Tetracyclic antidepressant, for neuropathic pain, 14

Tetrahydrocannabinol (THC), 33, 35f. See also Cannabinoids
nitrogen analog of, 39

Tetrahydrocannabivarin, 33

Thalamic syndromes, 8t

Thoracotomy, pain caused by, nerve block for, 49

Tiagabine, 27–28

Tizanidine
adverse effects and side effects of, 100
for cancer pain, 96t, 99–100
dosage and administration of, 99t

Tocainide, 49

Topical analgesics. See also specific drug
adjuvant, 71
advances in (future directions for), 71–72, 76–77
advantages of, 71
adverse effects and side effects of, 112
for cancer pain, 96t, 100
formulations of, 71
novel agents, 76–77
and oral analgesics, combination therapy with, 71, 76
pharmacology of, 112
for rheumatic pain, 109t, 112–113

Topiramate, 86
adverse effects and side effects of, 25t
for cancer pain, 96t
for cancer-related neuropathic pain, 101
contraindications to, 25t
dosage and administration of, 25t
indications for, 27
mechanism of action of, 10t, 25t
precautions with, 25t

Tramadol
adverse effects and side effects of, 83t, 84, 141
for chronic noncancer pain, 17
clomipramine and, drug-drug interactions, 138t
CYP2D6 inhibitors and, drug-drug interactions, 138t, 143
dosage and administration of, 83t, 84
imipramine and, drug-drug interactions, 138t
mechanism of action of, 10t, 83t
mirtazapine and, drug-drug interactions, 138t
for neuropathic pain, 15, 83t, 84
and other serotonergic agents, drug-drug interactions, 138t, 143
paroxetine and, drug-drug interactions, 138t
for phantom limb pain, 88
pharmacology of, 141
precautions with, 83t, 84
and serotonergic activity, 139t
and serotonin syndrome, 140–141
for spinal cord injury-related pain, 86–88
SSRIs and, drug-drug interactions, 138t
trazodone and, drug-drug interactions, 138t
and venlafaxine, comparison of, 141
venlafaxine and, drug-drug interactions, 138t, 141

Transcutaneous electrical nerve stimulation (TENS), 1

Transient receptor potential family of receptors, as drug target, 76, 85

Tranylcypromine, and serotonergic activity, 139t

Trazodone
and methadone, drug-drug interactions, 138t
and serotonergic activity, 139t
and tapentadol, drug-drug interactions, 138t
and tramadol, drug-drug interactions, 138t

Tricyclic antidepressants, 5, 9t, 11–13, 12t, 14. See also specific drug
adverse effects and side effects of, 18, 81t
analgesic effects of, dose and, 18
for cancer pain, 96t, 97–98
and carbamazepine, drug-drug interactions, 133t
for chronic noncancer pain, selection of, 17–19
dosage and administration of, 80
for fibromyalgia, 17, 109t, 110
for headache, 15–16
mechanism of action of, 80, 81t
molecular target of, 9t
for neuropathic pain, 14–15, 17, 80, 81t, 88–89
placebo-controlled trials of, 13t
and NSAIDs, drug-drug interactions, 135t, 143
and other serotonergic agents, drug-drug interactions, 143

Tricyclic antidepressants (Cont.)
patient education about, 18
and phenytoin, drug-drug interactions, 132t
precautions with, 81t
and serotonergic activity, 139t
and serotonin syndrome, 140
and SNRIs, drug-drug interactions, 132t
for spinal cord injury-related pain, 81t, 86–88
and SSRIs, drug-drug interactions, 132t
topical
  for cancer pain, 96t
  for rheumatic pain, 112
and venlafaxine, drug-drug interactions, 132t, 134t, 141
withdrawal of, 18
Trigeminal neuralgia, 79
carbamazepine for, 86
treatment of, 21, 23, 27
Trimipramine
adverse effects and side effects of, 12t
for arthritis pain, 16
dosage and administration of, 12t
half-life of, 12t
neurotransmitter profile of, 12 t
L-Tryptophan, and serotonergic activity, 139t

U

Ulnar nerve block, 48
Ultrasound, 1

V

Valproate, 28, 86
carbamazepine and, drug-drug interactions, 132t
Vanilloid receptor, subtype 1, as drug target, 9t, 75, 85
Venlafaxine, 11
adverse effects and side effects of, 12t, 81t, 141
and amitriptyline, drug-drug interactions, 141
for cancer pain, 96t, 98
dosage and administration of, 12t, 81t, 84
half-life of, 12t
for headache, 15–17
mechanism of action of, 81t
and methadone, drug-drug interactions, 138t, 141
for neuropathic pain, 14, 17, 80–84, 81t, 88
placebo-controlled trials of, 13t
neurotransmitter profile of, 12t
and NSAIDs, drug-drug interactions, 137t, 143
and other serotonergic agents, drug-drug interactions, 143
pharmacology of, 141
for postmastectomy pain, 88
for postoperative pain, dosage and administration of, 127t
precautions with, 81t
St. John's wort and, interactions between, 142t
and serotonergic activity, 139t
and serotonin syndrome, 140–141
and tapentadol, drug-drug interactions, 138t
and TCAs, drug-drug interactions, 132t, 134t, 141
and tramadol
  comparison of, 141
  drug-drug interactions, 138t, 141
Ventricular tachycardia, drug-induced, 18
Visceral pain, 8t
Vomiting. See Nausea and vomiting

W

Weight gain, drugs causing, 12t, 18
Withdrawal reaction(s), 16
World Health Organization (WHO), analgesic ladder/pain ladder, 2, 2f, 5–6, 6t
modifications of, 2–3

Y

Yoga, 1

Z

Zolendronate
for cancer pain, 97t
for cancer-related bone pain, 102–103
Zonisamide, 27–28
adverse effects and side effects of, 26t
contraindications to, 26t
dosage and administration of, 26t
mechanism of action of, 26t
precautions with, 26

www.ingramcontent.com/pod-product-compliance
Ingram Content Group UK Ltd.
Pitfield, Milton Keynes, MK11 3LW, UK
UKHW021258180426
11947UKWH00015B/905